WADA, the World Anti-Doping Agency

Examining the legitimacy of the World Anti-Doping Agency, this book offers a critical analysis of the anti-doping system and the social and behavioural processes that shape policy, asking why the current system is failing.

Featuring in-depth, contemporary case studies from around the world, including the whereabouts system, Lance Armstrong, therapeutic use exemptions, the Essendon Bombers, recreational drugs policy and the Russian Olympic doping programme, this is the first text to analyse empirically how the legitimacy of WADA is constructed, contested and managed in the field of anti-doping and the consequent impact this has on anti-doping. Based on the analysis of these case studies, the book discusses how legitimacy processes have shaped the current regulatory environment and offers structural and governance reforms to improve anti-doping policy design and implementation.

Adopting a unique theoretical perspective, rooted in a socio-cognitive perspective on organisational behaviour, this book is essential reading for any researcher or student working on drugs and doping in sport, sport management, the sociology of sport, governance, transnational organisations or strategic management. It also offers important insights for policymakers and administrators working in sport or in government.

Daniel Read is a lecturer in sport business at the Institute for Sport Business, Loughborough University London, United Kingdom.

James Skinner is a professor in sport business at the Institute for Sport Business, Loughborough University London, United Kingdom.

Daniel Lock is a principal academic in the Department of Sport and Event Management, Bournemouth University, United Kingdom.

Aaron CT Smith is a professor in sport business at the Institute for Sport Business, Loughborough University London, United Kingdom.

Routledge Research in Sport and Corruption

Series Editor: James Skinner
Loughborough University London, UK

Match-Fixing in Sport
Comparative Studies from Australia, Japan, Korea and Beyond
Edited by Stacey Steele and Hayden Opie

Corruption in Sport
Causes, Consequences, and Reform
Edited by Lisa A. Kihl

Restoring Trust in Sport
Corruption Cases and Solutions
Edited by Catherine Ordway

WADA, the World Anti-Doping Agency
A Multi-Level Legitimacy Analysis
Daniel Read, James Skinner, Daniel Lock and Aaron CT Smith

WADA, the World Anti-Doping Agency

A Multi-Level Legitimacy Analysis

Daniel Read, James Skinner, Daniel Lock, and Aaron CT Smith

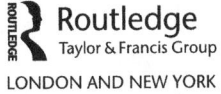
Routledge
Taylor & Francis Group
LONDON AND NEW YORK

First published 2021
by Routledge
2 Park Square, Milton Park, Abingdon, Oxon OX14 4RN

and by Routledge
605 Third Avenue, New York, NY 10017

Routledge is an imprint of the Taylor & Francis Group, an informa business

© 2021 Daniel Read, James Skinner, Daniel Lock and Aaron CT Smith

British Library Cataloguing-in-Publication Data
A catalogue record for this book is available from the British Library

Library of Congress Cataloging-in-Publication Data
Names: Read, Daniel, author. | Skinner, James, 1964- author. | Lock,
Daniel, author. | Smith, Aaron, 1972- author. | World Anti-Doping Agency.
Title: WADA, the world anti-doping agency : a multi-level legitimacy
analysis / Daniel Read, James Skinner, Daniel Lock, Aaron C.T. Smith.
Description: First. | Milton Park, Abingdon, Oxon ; New York NY :
Routledge, 2021. |
Series: Routledge research in sport and corruption | Includes
bibliographical references and index.
Identifiers: LCCN 2020050943 | ISBN 9780367540630 (hardback) | ISBN
9781003084297 (ebook)
Subjects: LCSH: Doping in sports. | Doping in sports--Political aspects.
Classification: LCC RC1230 .R42 2021 | DDC 362.29088/796--dc23
LC record available at https://lccn.loc.gov/2020050943

ISBN: 978-0-367-54063-0 (hbk)
ISBN: 978-0-367-54064-7 (pbk)
ISBN: 978-1-003-08429-7 (ebk)

Typeset in Goudy
by MPS Limited, Dehradun

Contents

Acknowledgements

Firstly, we would like to recognise all the academics and anti-doping professionals who have shared their feedback on the research that underpins this monograph over the past four years. Their thoughts have undoubtedly educated and guided our understanding and provided an insight into the reality of anti-doping management.

Secondly, we wish to acknowledge and thank Professor Bob Stewart and Dr Eric Schwarz (Victoria University, Australia) for their contribution to chapter Seven.

Finally, we would like to thank Loughborough University for providing the PhD funding that made this research possible.

List of Abbreviations

ADAMS	Anti-Doping Administration and Management System
ADRV	Anti-Doping Rule Violation
AFL	Australian Football League
ASADA	Australian Sports Anti-Doping Authority
BALCO	Bay Area Laboratory Co-Operative
BCCI	The Board of Control for Cricket in India
BOA	British Olympic Association
BWF	Bulgarian Weightlifting Federation
CAS	Court of Arbitration for Sport
CIRC	Cycling Independent Reform Commission
DCMS	Department for Digital, Culture, Media and Sport
EFC	Essendon Football Club
FIFA	International Federation of Association Football
FINA	International Federation of Swimming
IAAF	International Association of Athletics Federations
ICC	International Cricket Council
IF	International Federation
iNADO	Institute of National Anti-Doping Organisations
IOC	International Olympic Committee
ITA	International Testing Agency
ITF	International Tennis Federation
ISCCS	International Standard for Code Compliance by Signatories
LNDD	Laboratoire National de Détection du dopage
NADO	National Anti-Doping Organisation
OMADA	Olympic Movement Anti-Doping Agency
OOC	out-of-competition
PED	performance-enhancing drug
RUSADA	Russian Anti-Doping Agency
TUE	therapeutic use exemption
UCI	Union Cycliste Internationale
UEFA	Union of European Football Associations

UKAD	United Kingdom Anti-Doping Agency
USADA	United States Anti-Doping Agency
WADA	World Anti-Doping Agency
WADC	World Anti-Doping Code
WTA	World Tennis Association

Chapter 1

The current state of anti-doping

In his inaugural speech as the new president of the WADA, Witold Bańka reflected on the challenges the organisation has faced in recent years:

> On the one hand, these last years have tested the resolve and unity of the global anti-doping community like never before but they have also served as a catalyst to strengthen the system. And, they have demonstrated the persistent challenges of doping in sports, which calls for a dynamic approach and the financial means to get there.
>
> (WADA, 2020a, p. 15)

As WADA moves into its third decade as the chief regulator of anti-doping under the Olympic umbrella, Bańka's comment aptly positions the magnitude of the organisation's mission. Since its inception, WADA has expended most of its time and resources attenuating the impact of doping athletes, unruly signatories and, at times, the behaviour of its own staff. It is little surprise, then, that WADA's existence has been characterised by drama and scandal, given the cat-and-mouse nature of detecting doping in sport, the volatile geo-political forces that surround the Olympic Games ('Olympics' henceforth) and the media's love for the hero and villain narratives created by doping transgressions.

The poignant and significant question that emerges from this scenario is how WADA's handling of these challenges has impacted its various stakeholders, not least the athletes themselves. The way in which it has responded to the challenges presented has had significant ramifications for the current state of anti-doping policy and those to whom it applies. As we will examine in this book, WADA has long struggled with a lack of support from key stakeholders. Understanding how the dynamic relationship between WADA and its stakeholders has shaped policy presents significant learning opportunities for anti-doping practitioners, as well as the complex business of sports governance in general.

The concept of legitimacy, broadly understood as the perceived appropriateness of an organisation's behaviour, is relevant to understanding the relationship between WADA and its stakeholders. A commonly held argument in management science is that organisations perceived to be legitimate by their stakeholders are more likely to receive behavioural support and survive (Suchman, 1995). Accordingly, this book will use recent theoretical developments to examine the legitimacy of WADA in relation to two questions:

1.   How has WADA's legitimacy been challenged since its foundation?
2.   How has WADA responded to challenges to its legitimacy?

To explore these two questions, we present empirical findings from seven case studies of events and policies that have challenged the legitimacy of WADA. These case studies are: (1) the Lausanne Conference, (2) the whereabouts system, (3) Lance Armstrong and the International Cycling Union, (4) the therapeutic use exemptions system, (5) the Australian Football League (AFL) and Essendon Bombers case, (6) recreational drug prohibition and (7) the Russian Olympic doping scandal. These cases have been selected because they are high-profile, global issues that have occurred in the 20 years since WADA was founded.

Our analysis is premised on the observation that individuals or stakeholders evaluate organisations and their actions as objects. The degree to which individuals agree that an organisation's actions are appropriate (i.e., judgements of propriety) coalesce to reveal broader judgements of consensus or disagreement (i.e., the extent to which individuals agree or disagree about the legitimacy of an organisation). From our case analysis, we argue that WADA's legitimacy is unstable because stakeholders disagree about the legitimacy of the organisation and its policies.

From the case findings, we make three connected arguments. Firstly, the structure and design of the anti-doping system leads to conflict between stakeholders with different agendas. Secondly, the conflict between individuals and groups leads to decision-making by WADA that prioritises stakeholders that are most valuable to the organisation's legitimacy. Finally, prioritisation means that change and adaptation are limited to incremental shifts that maintain the current status quo rather than radical change. The implications of these arguments are significant because, unless it is able to reform, WADA will always struggle to develop consensus between stakeholders in order to achieve its stated goal of doping-free sport. From this position, we conclude with a series of reform suggestions to address the legitimacy issues raised by the organisation's design and policies.

The remainder of this chapter will examine WADA's progress and effectiveness in regulating anti-doping efforts and achieving its ambition of doping-free sport. Using anti-doping network development, anti-doping testing statistics and anti-doping policy harmonisation as outcome measures, it is concluded that WADA has struggled – and still struggles – to achieve its goals because of a lack of behavioural support from stakeholders. Therefore, studying WADA's legitimacy becomes crucial to understanding its lack of progress towards doping-free sport. Before examining the current progress of anti-doping, it is instructive to examine the history of doping that led to the formation of WADA to situate the organisation's progress against previous anti-doping efforts.

The emergence of WADA

Doping refers to the use of prohibited performance-enhancing drugs (PED) and techniques to gain a competitive advantage in sport. The use of PED is not unique to contemporary sport. One of the earliest examples of a prohibitory drug policy in sport occurred in 1889 when doping of horses for competitive gain led to bans due to concerns about gambling (Gleaves, 2012). Despite this early example, the implementation of sporting anti-doping policy in the 20th century was seen as slow and, arguably, ineffective (Houlihan, 2002a). At the same time, doping in sport increased in complexity from a typically individual behaviour to a collective behaviour that often involves a network of different stakeholders including athletes, support staff, coaches, sports administrators and even international drug-trafficking cartels.

The history of sport is littered with cases of socially organised doping (Waddington & Møller, 2019) orchestrated by members of teams and nations. *Socially organised doping* refers to networks of interaction used by a team or nation to enable doping. There are various examples, which include the Olympic doping programme, operated by the German Democratic Republic in the 1970s and 1980s and the concealment of positive drug tests given by US Olympic athletes in the 1990s (Christie, 2003). These examples are distinctive because they suggest deeper cultures of drug use led and managed at an organisational or governmental level. Furthermore, detection usually relies on non-analytical anti-doping rule violations (ADRVs). These are violations proven by evidence other than a positive test, such as possession of PED or doping paraphernalia. However, it took until 1998 and the Festina Scandal at the Tour de France to set the conditions for the creation of an international anti-doping organisation.

The Festina Scandal represented a turning point in anti-doping policy. French customs officials arrested professional cycling team managers, soigneurs (support staff responsible for cyclists' well-being) and medical staff for the possession and administration of PED at the Tour de France. The scandal demonstrated widespread PED use in cycling and almost ended the Tour de France (Kamber, 2011). As a result of cycling's Olympic status, the failings of its anti-doping policy also meant that the International Olympic Committee (IOC) was scrutinised by governments that were concerned with doping violations and approaches to discourage anti-doping through policy development (e.g., Norway, Canada, United Kingdom). Hanstad, Smith, and Waddington (2008) argued that to keep control of anti-doping policy, the IOC strategically arranged the First Conference on Doping in Sport (hereinafter called the Lausanne Conference) in order to suggest the establishment of an Olympic Movement Anti-Doping Agency for the oversight of sports governed by the IOC. These proposals were rejected, as government representatives used the conference to criticise the IOC's general lack of concern for integrity in sports following the Salt-Lake City bidding scandal (Wenn, Barney, & Martyn, 2011) and specific failure to effectively regulate anti-doping (Hanstad et al., 2008). The outcome of the Lausanne Conference was a compromised agreement to develop an independent international anti-doping organisation responsible for regulating drugs in sport. This organisation was to be funded equally by the IOC and national governments globally relative to their gross domestic product. In November 1999, WADA was created with the mandate to coordinate and harmonise the international effort to stop doping in sport (Houlihan, 2002a).

WADA aims to create 'a world where all athletes can compete in a doping free sporting environment' via its primary purpose of harmonizing anti-doping policies in all sports and all countries (WADA, 2020b). Although a non-governmental organisation in form, WADA's underpinning positioning has been variously conceptualised as a hybrid organisation (Wagner, 2009), a cross-sector social partnership (Toohey & Beaton, 2017) and a multi-lateral regime (Skinner, Read, & Kihl, 2017) among others. For clarity, and consistent with previous arguments (Gray, 2019; Houlihan, 2014; Skinner et al., 2017), we take the position that WADA should be perceived as the focal organisation of a larger regime, as it unifies sporting and political authorities towards a common goal of doping-free sport by creating general agreements on appropriate behaviour through policy (Krasner, 1983; Thompson & Verdier, 2014). WADA then seeks to achieve its anti-doping mission through multiple aspects of the regime.

WADA consists of a 14-member Executive Committee and a 38-member Foundation Board, both of which are equally composed of state government authorities and Olympic movement representatives, in addition to technical staff (e.g., human resources). Notably, WADA is funded by equivalent contributions from the IOC (50%) and national governments (50%, divided unequally between individual and national contributions). The regime is also enacted through the rules and policies of the World Anti-Doping Code (WADC), a living policy document that sets out the responsibilities for different stakeholders in relation to anti-doping. Sport organisations that can become signatories to the WADC include international federations (IFs), national Olympic committees and multi-sport organisations, and in doing so, agree to implement and comply with the policies laid out in the document. The regime further consists of the UNESCO International Convention against Doping in Sport, which enables state governments to officially signify their recognition of the rules and requirements spelt out in the WADC. Anti-doping testing and management are then delegated to National Anti-Doping Organisations (NADOs), IFs and mega-event organisers such as the IOC. Through these series of partnerships and documentation, the WADA regime was formed, and WADA (the organisation) sits at the nexus as the global regulator of signatory compliance with the WADC. The centralisation of anti-doping compliance and governance, in theory, removed the previous conflicts of interest that plagued IFs simultaneously policing and promoting sport, characteristic of the period prior to WADA, thereby setting the foundations for effective anti-doping control.

New regime, same problems?

Despite the creation of the WADA regime, numerous high-profile examples of socially organised doping punctuate the authority's existence. For example, the Bay Area Laboratory Co-operative scandal in 2003 occurred because a syringe of a designer steroid was anonymously provided to investigators. In turn, this piece of evidence implicated dozens of athletes in various Olympic and professional sports. In 2006, a raid by Italian police uncovered PED and doping paraphernalia belonging to six Austrian Winter Olympians, who received life bans for doping, despite having never given a positive sample. Lance Armstrong and the U.S. Postal Service Cycling team operated a doping programme that yielded seven consecutive Tour de France general classification victories from 1999 to 2005. In 2015, evidence emerged of a socially organised doping programme in Russia, involving over 1,000 summer and winter Olympic athletes at the London 2012 and Sochi 2014 Olympics. As recently as February 2019, Operation Aderlass exposed a multi-sport network of European athletes involved in blood doping. These examples reveal that athletes were able to avoid detection via traditional testing methods and were only caught because of information provided by whistle-blowers.

The fact that doping operations reminiscent of the Festina Affair and the East German system are still feasible 20 years after the creation of WADA provides justification for examining the progress and effectiveness of the organisation. In addition to the uncovering of socially organised doping, there are further reasons to assess the progress of WADA. Firstly, WADA receives approximately US$18 million per year of public funding from around the world, and an account of its appropriate and effective expenditure is warranted. Secondly, sport is important to many nations because it is used as a tool for social development and physical well-being. Doping can be constructed as a threat to such social values. Thirdly, some critics argue that prohibiting all drugs in sport is unachievable (e.g., Kayser & Smith, 2008). Therefore, understanding the tractability of the problem is a key practical concern. Fourthly, anti-doping policy infringes on athletes' human rights and can be justified only if the system works (Dimeo & Møller, 2018). Fifthly, anti-doping is designed to protect athletes from misusing potentially harmful substances; therefore, the effectiveness of the system has significant implications for athlete welfare. Finally, if organisations are involved in doping activities (e.g., facilitation or provision of doping), all athletes and organisations that comply with anti-doping requirements are disadvantaged. Acknowledging these reasons alongside the recurrent exposure of socially organised doping, there is justification in this chapter's ambition to assess the progress WADA has made in achieving doping-free sport. The resulting analysis helps to understand the challenges faced by WADA in achieving its lofty ambitions.

The progress of WADA

To evaluate the progress of the WADA regime in harmonising anti-doping policy between WADC signatories and its aim of doping-free sport, we draw on multiple indicators of success. Houlihan and Hanstad (2019) have previously assessed WADA's performance (outputs) and effectiveness (outcomes) in comparison to other regimes through an examination of internal (e.g., organisational design) and contextual factors (e.g., scientific developments). They concluded that WADA's ability to create outputs, such as the UNESCO Agreement, is impressive given its available resources. However, WADA's outputs have not translated into the reduction of doping in sport. Acknowledging that there are limitations to studying regime outcomes (i.e., behavioural change of athletes and signatories) of anti-doping under WADA primarily due to accurately measuring and interpreting doping rates and monitoring compliance, alternative regime outcome measures are considered. These outcome measures are: (1) the development of a global anti-doping network; (2) anti-doping testing statistics; and (3) implementation of the WADC. These measures are used as we argue they provide a balanced, multi-dimensional perspective of WADA's progress towards its aim of doping-free sport. When considering all three outcome measures, it is apparent that WADA has made little progress towards its goal of 'doping-free' sport.

Anti-doping network development

WADA's ability to develop a global anti-doping network to enact the WADC is an indication of its intention to change the behaviour of stakeholders in accordance with anti-doping policy. Toohey and Beaton (2017) asserted that WADA's ability to establish a global anti-doping network between conflicting and unconcerned stakeholders is evidence of the organisation's progress. Houlihan (2002a) noted that the establishment of WADA created stability in the anti-doping regime between previously fragmented actors such as IFs and governments. Furthermore, Houlihan (2014), stated that the creation and ongoing review of the WADC is the most prominent success of WADA in developing the criteria for anti-doping policy in testing, management and the sanctioning of athletes and organisations. Coupled with its acceptance by 660 signatories globally, this means that, in principle, all signatories to the WADC should be operating anti-doping procedures aligned with WADA's guidance. These signatories form a global network through which the WADA regime seeks to regulate anti-doping.

Jedlicka and Hunt (2013) pointed to the creation of the UNESCO International Convention against Doping in Sport in 2005 as a key juncture in the legal establishment of WADA. The UNESCO Convention was designed to formalise government involvement in anti-doping management by aligning domestic legal practice with the WADC. This is an example of WADA's success in establishing and growing a network of national governments, as the UNESCO Convention on doping became the most quickly ratified Convention in UNESCO history (Houlihan, 2014). Kamber (2011) and Houlihan (2009) also concluded that the establishment of WADA has led to positive progress in anti-doping management and policy at a national level, such as the development of a network of NADOs globally. Specific to network development, Houlihan and Hanstad (2019) concluded that WADA has engaged several significant stakeholders, such as governments and transnational law enforcement organisations, into the anti-doping network.

From an anti-doping network development perspective, the growth in the number of signatories under WADA regulation is a positive outcome of the regime. WADA has positioned itself as the central system of government responsible for the regulation of anti-doping and, in doing so, created pathways to enact change in anti-doping practices. From this perspective the WADA regime has made significant progress towards PED-free sport. However, the Olympic Charter (IOC, 2019) stipulates that sports organisations must become a signatory to WADA for Olympic recognition. This coercion confounds the degree to which network growth has occurred through free choice or a belief that anti-doping is important. Furthermore, given the complex antecedents of doping, the diversity and power of stakeholders involved and the behavioural change required, network developments alone are insufficient to achieve doping-free sport. Therefore, evaluating network development against the additional regime outcome measures of anti-doping testing statistics and harmonisation of anti-doping policy enables further reflection on progress.

Anti-doping testing statistics

WADA's progress towards doping-free sport can also be examined using drug testing statistics. The most recent data from 2018 demonstrates that the number of athletes being tested is steadily increasing. Likewise, the number of blood tests supporting an athlete's biological passport (a record of an athlete's various haematological values over time such as red blood cells), which is thought to be more effective than single tests in detecting blood doping, has increased, which is a positive sign of engagement. Meanwhile, the rate of adverse analytical findings (AAF) has decreased from a meagre 1.43% (4,596) in 2017 to 1.42% (4,896) in 2018. The AAF percentages do not show how many athletes were eventually sanctioned for a demonstrable ADRV. Nor do these figures reveal the percentage of athletes who produced an AAF, as multiple tests may be required per athlete in systems such as the athlete biological passport. These analytical findings suggest an underwhelmingly low incidence of positive tests and call into question the significant financial investment in the anti-doping system. It could be argued that the AAF figures show doping is not prevalent in sport, however, when compared to estimates of PED use, the more likely explanation is that testing is not detecting the true extent of doping.

Researchers have estimated that the proportion of athletes using PED ranges from 14% to 39% depending on the sport (De Hon, Kuipers, & van Bottenburg, 2015). There are methodological concerns about the validity of self-report measures used to estimate doping rates. As a result, supplemental testing procedures such as randomised response techniques have been considered. Randomised response technique is a survey method that requires participants to first complete a random task or question (e.g., flipping a coin), the outcome of which is unknown to the researcher. Depending on the outcome of this task, the participant is informed to answer the question about the sensitive topic truthfully or with a predetermined answer regardless of the truth. The researcher then has no idea if an individual has answered truthfully or not but can calculate an overall value for the group from the amount expected to have answered truthfully, based on the randomness of the first task (e.g., 50% honest, 50% predetermined using a coin flip). This technique is a promising method to assess with greater accuracy doping rates as it promotes confidentiality. Ulrich et al. (2018) used a randomised response technique with 2,167 international standard athletics competitors across two competitions in order to guarantee anonymity. Their results indicated that between 43.6% and 57.1% of athletes had doped in the past year, and these figures may be even higher due to the unwillingness of participants to admit doping behaviour. Elbe and Pitsch (2018) used the same methodology with 771 Danish athletes, estimating previous season doping rates between 22.6% and 35.7%. Taken together, randomised response technique estimates significantly exceed the 1.42–1.43% of AAF reported. Qualitative studies have also supported the assertion that doping in certain sports is perceived to be widespread, and as a necessary condition for success (Engelberg, Moston, & Skinner, 2015; Kirby, Moran, & Guerin, 2011; Ohl, Fincoeur, Lentillon-Kaestner, Defrance, & Brissonneau, 2015). Therefore, athletes are not deterred by anti-doping policy, do not have a choice about doping or consider the benefits of doping to outweigh the costs of being caught. All three scenarios suggest that WADA and the WADC are currently failing to achieve behavioural support from athletes and doping-free sport.

The claim that WADA has struggled to modify athlete behaviour is corroborated by evidence that athletes perceive the WADC to be unfairly implemented. For example, Bloodworth and McNamee (2010) found that British athletes were sceptical about the rigour of anti-doping testing in other nations. Similarly, using a sample of elite Danish athletes, Overbye (2016) found that 85% of athletes thought that 'doping control is downgraded in certain countries because medals have higher priority', and 46% of athletes perceived that 'doping control in other countries is sometimes so unprofessional that it is possible to cheat' (p. 12). Using the same sample of Danish athletes, Overbye and Wagner (2014) found a similar distrust in how the whereabouts system (the requirement for elite athletes to provide a daily time and location to enable unannounced anti-doping testing) operates in countries outside of Denmark. Efverström, Ahmadi, Hoff, and Bäckström (2016) found that in a sample of 261 athletes from 51 nations, 44% were suspicious of anti-doping systems in other countries. Qualitative studies have found similar distrust among athletes in the harmonisation of anti-doping policy implementation (Efverström, Bäckström, Ahmadi, & Hoff, 2016; Henning & Dimeo, 2019). The analyses presented in these studies support the idea of anti-doping, but question the practical application (Efverström et al., 2016; Henning & Dimeo, 2019; Overbye, 2016). It appears that athletes perceive discrepancies in anti-doping policy implementation internationally, which undermines support for WADA from the group it primarily serves (Woolway, Lazuras, Barkoukis, & Petróczi, 2020).

Further evidence that high estimates of doping in sport are the consequences of a lack of behavioural support emerges from athlete perceptions of the testing system. Detection reflects athlete perceptions about the likelihood of being caught, while deterrents refer to how athletes perceive the outcomes of being detected. The assumption that increasing the likelihood of detection and the severity of deterrents will reduce undesired behaviours, although popular in many aspects of public criminal justice, lacks supporting evidence (Pratt, Cullen, Blevins, Daigle, & Madensen, 2006). It is similarly problematic in relation to anti-doping (Moston, Engelberg, & Skinner, 2015; Strelan & Boeckmann, 2006). Research supports arguments that generally athletes (1) do not perceive the likelihood of being selected for testing as a deterrent to doping (Henning & Dimeo, 2019; Overbye, 2016), (2) do not perceive that they will be selected for testing (Engelberg et al., 2015; Overbye, Knudsen, & Pfister, 2013), and/or (3) do not perceive that more testing increases their chance of being detected (Baudouin & Szymanski, 2016). Evidence also supports the assertion that a ban from competition is generally seen as a deterrent, but a financial sanction may be a greater deterrent (Overbye, Elbe, Knudsen, & Pfister, 2015), as are improved diagnostics (Westmattelmann, Dreiskämper, Strauß, Schewe, & Plass, 2018). Yet these findings present a scenario that is concerning for the WADC which was grounded in detection and deterrence principles.

The combined presence of drug testing and low positive detection rates should not be assumed as evidence that a sport does not have a problem with PED use. The numerous retrospective cases of athletes passing tests who were later shown to be doping support that tests are not foolproof. For instance, Lance Armstrong is reported to have been tested between 260 and 600 times in his career (Austen, 2012) but avoided detection through scientific and pragmatic tactics. Like many other cases, whistle-blowers were ultimately responsible for his detection. WADA's establishment of an international network of anti-doping stakeholders as a regime outcome indicates positive progress towards doping-free sport, but analysis of testing statistics suggests a lack of progress. It is apparent that there are problems in gaining behavioural support from athletes that may be due to perceived inequalities in testing globally as well as perceptions that they are unlikely to be caught. Given the inequities in testing, the following section will analyse the implementation of the WADC globally to further understand WADA's progress towards doping-free sport.

Implementation of the World Anti-Doping Code

WADA states that it aims to bring consistency to anti-doping policy (i.e., harmonisation) as one of the main ways of achieving doping-free sport. Therefore, it is appropriate to evaluate the implementation of, and compliance with, the WADC when assessing progress. Compliance relates to the *depth* of WADC implementation and is monitored on factors such as the number of tests conducted annually (Hanstad & Houlihan, 2015). Purposeful decisions were made in the phrasing of the WADC to allow interpretation in implementing anti-doping policy to account for differences between nations (e.g., cultural, political, financial) at the sacrifice of specificity and transparency (Houlihan, 2002b). Consequently, compliance with the regime has been a problem for WADA (Houlihan, 2014). Additionally, comparing the problems faced by WADA with other international regimes, Gray (2019) suggested that compliance issues in top-down regimes stem from the dependence upon signatories. Hanstad and Houlihan (2015) advocated bilateral agreements between established and developing NADOs, such as Norway and China, as a viable strategy to improve anti-doping compliance. However, bilateral agreements require willingness from less compliant NADOs, and the flexibility in the WADC means that organisations without the motivation to fully enforce anti-doping policy need to commit only to a shallow level of compliance (Houlihan, 2014).

Indeed, there is evidence that the introduction of the WADC has led to an unequal implementation of policy. For instance, the results of a survey of 32 NADOs in 2010 showed only 23 had a registered testing pool for the whereabouts system, a protocol crucial for out-of-competition (OOC) testing (Hanstad, Skille, & Loland, 2010). Significantly, the analysis showed that traditional explanations of poor compliance such as lack of resources (operationalised by budget), or capacity (operationalised by staff size), did not predict variations. Based on the available evidence, depth of compliance remains an issue for WADA. In its 2019 Compliance Strategy for strengthening signatory anti-doping programmes, WADA concedes, 'Different Signatories have evolved at varying paces resulting in significant differences in compliance capabilities amongst Signatories' (WADA, 2019, p. 4).

Hanstad et al. (2010) summarised the problem of varying compliance: 'The fact that athletes in different countries are treated differently by their NADOs regarding sanctions is, it may be argued, detrimental to the legitimacy and sense of fairness of anti-doping' (p. 426). Variations in compliance are attributable to several factors, which impact how the progress of WADA can be assessed, and therefore require exploration. In reviewing the challenges for gaining compliance with the WADC, Houlihan (2002b, 2014) divided potential reasons into inability, inadvertence and choice. These categories provide a useful conceptual tool to structure existing research into the harmonisation issues WADA faces.

Inability

Inability refers to a lack of financial and technical resources, which lead to incorrect implementation of the WADC (e.g., Hanstad et al., 2010; Houlihan, 2002b; Kustec Lipicer, & McArdle, 2014). Pound, Ayotte, Parkinson, Pengilly, and Ryan (2013) has acknowledged that some signatories are under-resourced and there may be discrepancies between WADA-certified laboratories due to differences in technical resources. Some critics have extended this argument to suggest that the demanding financial burdens of the WADC purposefully ensure that international sporting success remains within the so-called first world or global north (Henne, 2014; Park, 2005). Compliance issues due to financial inability are exemplified in developing nations where governments must prioritise funding more essential societal needs such as healthcare, infrastructure and sanitation (WADA, 2020c). Although a lack of resources may be a valid reason in some situations, it also provides a veil for nations and sporting organisations that do not share the same cultural values around anti-doping in sport (Gray, 2019). Additionally, sponsors, leagues and non-profit international sports governing bodies, such as the IOC, possess significant financial capital that could be used to address implementation issues attributed to a lack of resources.

Inadvertence

Inadvertence is a potential outcome of the deliberate flexibility and vagueness of the WADC. In trying to allow for differences between members, direct guidance is compromised (Houlihan, 2002b, 2014). Research with elite athletes highlighted discrepancies in anti-doping testing conditions between different national and cultural contexts (Efverström et al., 2016; Henning & Dimeo, 2019). Without data from those responsible for implementing policy, it is hard to determine if these differences are due to inability, inadvertence or choice, but it does confirm that interpretive flexibility in the WADC has real-world implications for harmonisation. Wagner and Hanstad (2011) suggested that there is merit in the argument that culturally based interpretations of the WADC influence implementation, even between culturally similar countries.

The inability of WADA to control legal proceedings within countries and ensure harmony between outcomes of similar cases across nations also creates inequities (Henne 2014; Møller, 2016). WADA can appeal signatory decisions to the Court of Arbitration for Sport (CAS) if it believes that the WADC has not been implemented correctly. Yet CAS is not without criticism as the evidentiary approach it takes differs from that of other tribunals (Mahoney, 2018), introducing yet another layer of potential discrepancy in WADC implementation. Hanstad and Houlihan (2015) discussed an interesting case of inadvertence in their case study of bilateral collaboration between Norway, a country with an established NADO, and China, a country developing an anti-doping programme.

Through collaboration focused on sharing information, China has developed its system and depth of compliance. However, much like inability, the problem with inadvertence is how to identify honest and deliberate cases that are disguised as inadvertence.

Choice

The final category is *choice*, which is a deliberate rather than unintended decision by an organisation to deviate from the WADC. This antecedent to compliance issues has received the greatest attention from researchers and commentators (Duval, 2016; Haugen & Popela, 2015; Houlihan, 2014; Houlihan & Hanstad, 2019; Pound et al., 2013). Research exploring choice as a reason for compliance issues can be divided into social and procedural factors. Social factors are reasons that may initially motivate the choice to avoid compliance, while procedural factors are features of the anti-doping regime that make avoiding compliance more favourable.

Social factors

We conceptualise social factors as reasons that organisations may not prioritise anti-doping, therefore leading to a lack of harmonisation. An often-cited WADA working group report (Pound et al., 2013) into the lack of effectiveness of testing programmes provides a clear indication that social issues exist, stating that 'the real problems are the human and political factors. There is no general appetite to undertake the effort and expense of a successful effort to deliver doping free sport' (p. 3). Although the report is seven years old at the time of writing this book, the argument is as valid now as it was then.

WADA regulates members from different cultures (both organisationally and culturally). Although the WADC has flexibility to allow for regional differences in resources, it still applies moral cultural beliefs to different contexts (Tamburrini, 2006). From Tamburrini's perspective, other cultures might not perceive anti-doping in sport as prominently as the Anglo-Saxon nations primarily behind the creation of WADA (Houlihan & Hanstad, 2019), but rather as a prerequisite to participation. In this situation, shallow compliance bestows access to elite sport without changing fundamental beliefs, especially if compliance monitoring is superficial. For example, Hong (2006) emphasised that China has made great progress towards anti-doping policy, but the social, economic and cultural factors around drug use in Chinese sport mean that there is still a great incentive for sport administrators, coaches and athletes to cheat. China is one example of a country where the motivation to be compliant may not stem from a deep-rooted belief in anti-doping, but in a desire to host mega sporting events (Tan, Bairner, & Chen, 2020). Opposingly, Gilberg, Breivik, and Loland (2006) found widespread negative perceptions of doping in Norwegian culture, a nation leading anti-doping efforts (Skille, Hanstad, & Tjernsbekk, 2011). Considering these cases, there is evidence to support cultural explanations of shallow compliance and a lack of harmonisation.

The public importance of anti-doping within sport has become further institutionalised in WADA's lifetime, creating pressure on national Olympic committees and sporting organisations to engage with anti-doping policy (Hanstad & Houlihan, 2015; Skille et al., 2011; Toohey & Beaton, 2017; Wagner 2010). Failure to do so implies a lack of concern with the issue. Furthermore, the IOC stipulates that IFs and national Olympic committees are expected to 'adopt and implement the World Anti-Doping Code' (IOC, 2019). These pressures placed on sporting organisations need to be considered against the ongoing commercialisation, politicisation, and professionalisation of sport (Grix & Carmichael, 2012; Hoye, Smith, Nicholson, & Stewart, 2015). These processes have inflated power asymmetries as central funding bodies, high-profile sponsors and audio-visual rights holders now dominate sport, and gaining support from such powerful audiences is an integral strategy to achieve profit maximisation and survival (Robinson, 2015). Problematically, anti-doping policy may be detrimental to performance quality and national success, as catching cheats and exposing doping may exclude a nation's top athletes, reduce competition quality, deter sponsors and create a negative image of a sport. Therefore, the human and political factors that Pound et al. (2013) identifies, and which underpin ineffectiveness, are still present.

Procedural factors

The central procedural factor explaining why nations and organisations may choose to avoid full compliance is WADA's lack of disciplinary power. Until recently, WADA could only judge nations as non-compliant, but required signatories such as the IOC to determine and impose penalties. In reviewing the Russian systematic doping programme, Duval (2016) suggested that to compensate, WADA must prioritise compliance monitoring and investigatory strategies. Similarly, Houlihan's (2014) analysis showed that WADA should monitor depth of compliance rather than simple implementation indicators. The introduction of the International Standard for Code Compliance by Signatories in 2018 stipulated a clear graded system of punishments that WADA can implement to signatories deemed non-compliant. Other researchers have gone further to suggest that nations and sporting organisations should bear economic consequences for doping to dissuade them from non-compliance (Maennig, 2014; Mazanov & Connor, 2010). Until a suitable solution is identified, countries that choose superficial compliance undermine the goal of harmonisation.

A more complex factor is the inherent conflicts of interest within the WADA regime (Haugen & Popela, 2015) and its executive body (Eber, 2002). Conflict within the Executive Committee and Foundation Board should be considered a procedural factor. Using economic modelling, Eber (2002) demonstrated that WADA was destined to fail if it did not establish a leader who was 'insensitive to the economic value of the sport' (p. 94), or who incentivised the president to maximise anti-doping efforts. Eber concluded that WADA executives may try to protect the economic value of sport if they have other roles in sport. The outcome is that compliance issues may appear more favourable because those with an economic or political stake in sport may act to make punishments less severe. This factor is related to WADA's previous inability to dispense penalties. For example, despite WADA advocating a blanket ban on all Russian athletes at the Rio Olympics, the IOC deferred this decision to IFs. Only a few sports, however, chose to enact such a severe penalty. Notwithstanding, WADA is aware that the Executive Committee members hold dual responsibilities to organisations with commercial and performance motives and have since stipulated that WADA's president and vice-president must not have any other roles with a sport organisation. They have also created positions for independent members of the Executive Committee, but the problem of conflict remains unresolved.

There is also concern about the conflict of interest that results from sport organisations simultaneously promoting and policing sport. WADA is a regulatory body and is only responsible for developing and monitoring the implementation of the WADC; signatories are responsible for implementation. Therefore, signatories simultaneously pursue organisational goals (e.g., competitive success, revenue generation, greater participation rates) and enact anti-doping policy, which has the potential to harm these objectives. Using economic modelling, Haugen and Popela (2015) demonstrated that there are financial incentives for sports administrators to not only condemn but also tolerate doping in sport to a certain extent as it may increase spectator demand. This is because PED use can improve competition quality and the likelihood of record-breaking performances which attract fans. The formation of the International Testing Agency in 2018 may have reduced the conflict between policing and promoting sport by outsourcing anti-doping. However, its success is dependent on the resources of the organisation it is working on behalf of. NADOs may also be subject to pressures to ease anti-doping procedures. Nations using sport as a tool for national promotion have little incentive to comply as anti-doping may prohibit top athletes from competition (Houlihan & Preece, 2007; Kamber, 2011). This issue bridges social and procedural factors as the current design of the anti-doping system renders it possible for members to pursue their own agendas, demonstrating the complex underpinnings of compliance problems.

In summary, one of WADA's primary strategies towards achieving doping-free sport is ensuring harmonised local implementation of the WADC globally. The progress of WADA in harmonising anti-doping regulation and achieving its goal of doping-free sport has been undermined by social and procedural factors. The conflicting pressures placed on signatories to the WADC, WADA's lack of effective monitoring systems and flexibility in the WADC mean that signatories can avoid anti-doping responsibilities. In doing so, signatories create a space in which athletes are not deterred from doping, perceive that they are able to dope without fear of detection and assume that their opponents are free to dope due to inequalities in testing between nations.

WADA's progress to date

Complementary to Houlihan and Hanstad (2019), the three outcome measures used to evaluate the progress of WADA (network development, testing and implementation) suggested that a lack of behavioural support from WADC signatories is the primary challenge to WADA's goal of doping-free sport. Despite making positive progress towards the development of a global anti-doping network, WADA has struggled to gain behavioural support from athletes, potentially due to a perceived lack of deterrents and unequal testing. These factors can be attributed to signatory compliance issues with the WADC. The lack of behavioural support from signatories to fully engage with the WADC due to inability, inadvertence or choice appears to be a critical issue in explaining the ineffectiveness of WADA to create doping-free sport. Understanding the social pressures within the field of sport and anti-doping that influence the behavioural support of signatories towards WADA is central to improving the anti-doping system.

Institutional theory proposes that organisational behaviour is more complex than rational decision-making and includes a social component that pressures organisations to behave in a manner perceived to be 'legitimate' regardless of whether this helps or harms technical efficiency (DiMaggio & Powell, 1983; Meyer & Rowan, 1977; Suchman, 1995; Zucker, 1977). Consequently, understanding the relationship between WADA's legitimacy, its signatories and other stakeholders is integral to understanding WADA's progress in creating doping-free sport. We use institutional theory, and multi-level legitimacy theory specifically (Bitektine & Haack, 2015; Suchman, 1995), as a theoretical lens to understand why WADA suffers from a lack of behavioural support from signatories. By using multiple case studies of issues that have challenged WADA's legitimacy, the aim of this book is to analyse the legitimacy of WADA from a multi-level legitimacy perspective. Taking the next step in our elaboration and interrogation of WADA's legitimacy, chapter two outlines institutional theory, provides a detailed discussion of multi-level legitimacy theories relevance to WADA and describes data sources underpinning the ensuing cases.

Following on from chapter two, case studies of the Lausanne Conference, the whereabouts system, Lance Armstrong and the International Cycling Union, the therapeutic use exemption system, the Essendon Bombers scandal, the prohibition of recreational substances and the Russian Olympic doping scandal are presented in chapters three to nine. The analysis presented in these case studies demonstrates the complex nature of WADA's legitimacy and relationships with different stakeholders. Chapter ten then examines the insight from these cases to argue that WADA's legitimacy will always remain highly contested unless there is significant change in the structures, processes and functioning of anti-doping. This position goes on to inform clear recommendations for change.

References

Austen, I., (2012). Report Describes How Armstrong and His Team Eluded Doping Tests. https://www.nytimes.com/.

Baudouin, C., & Szymanski, S. (2016). Testing the testers: Do more tests deter athletes from doping? *International Journal of Sport Finance, 11*(4), 349–363.

Bitektine, A., & Haack, P. (2015). The 'macro' and the 'micro' of legitimacy: Toward a multilevel theory of the legitimacy process. *Academy of Management Review, 40*(1), 49–75.

Bloodworth, A., & McNamee, M. (2010). Clean Olympians? Doping and anti-doping: The views of talented young British athletes. *International Journal of Drug Policy, 21*(4), 276–282.

Christie, J. (2003). U.S. hid failed tests, files reveal. *The Globe and Mail.* Retrieved from https://www.theglobeandmail.com/.

De Hon, O., Kuipers, H., & van Bottenburg, M. (2015). Prevalence of doping use in elite sports: A review of numbers and methods. *Sports Medicine, 45*(1), 57–69.

DiMaggio, P., & Powell, W.W. (1983). The iron cage revisited: Collective rationality and institutional isomorphism in organizational fields. *American Sociological Review, 48*(2), 147–160.

Dimeo, P., & Møller, V. (2018). *The anti-doping crisis in sport: Causes, consequences, solutions.* London, UK: Routledge.

Duval, A. (2016). *Tackling doping seriously – Reforming the world anti-doping system after the Russian scandal.* Lausanne, Switzerland: ASSER Policy Brief.

Eber, N. (2002). Credibility and independence of the World Anti-Doping Agency: A Barro-Gordon-type approach to antidoping policy. *Journal of Sports Economics, 3*(1), 90–96.

Efverström, A., Ahmadi, N., Hoff, D., & Bäckström, Å. (2016). Anti-doping and legitimacy: An international survey of elite athletes' perceptions. *International Journal of Sport Policy and Politics, 8*(3), 491–514.

Efverström, A., Bäckström, Å., Ahmadi, N., & Hoff, D. (2016). Contexts and conditions for a level playing field: Elite athletes' perspectives on anti-doping in practice. *Performance Enhancement & Health, 5*(2), 77–85.

Elbe, A.M., & Pitsch, W. (2018). Doping prevalence among Danish elite athletes. *Performance Enhancement & Health, 6*(1), 28–32.

Engelberg, T., Moston, S., & Skinner, J. (2015). The final frontier of anti-doping: A study of athletes who have committed doping violations. *Sport Management Review, 18*(2), 268–279.

Gilberg, R., Breivik, G., & Loland, S. (2006). Anti-doping in sport: The Norwegian perspective. *Sport in Society, 9*(2), 334–353.

Gleaves, J. (2012). Enhancing the odds: Horse racing, gambling and the first anti-doping movement in sport, 1889–1911. *Sport in History, 32*(1), 26–52.

Gray, S. (2019). Achieving compliance with the World Anti-Doping Code: Learning from the implementation of another international agreement. *International Journal of Sport Policy and Politics, 11*(2), 247–260.

Grix, J., & Carmichael, F. (2012). Why do governments invest in elite sport? A polemic. *International Journal of Sport Policy and Politics, 4,* 73–90. 10.1080/19406940.2011.627358.

Hanstad, D., & Houlihan, B. (2015). Strengthening global anti-doping policy through bilateral collaboration: The example of Norway and China. *International Journal of Sport Policy and Politics, 7*(4), 587–604.

Hanstad, D.V., Skille, E.Å., & Loland, S. (2010). Harmonization of anti-doping work: Myth or reality? *Sport in Society, 13*(3), 418–430.

Hanstad, D.V., Smith, A., & Waddington, I. (2008). The establishment of the World Anti-Doping Agency: A study of the management of organizational change and unplanned outcomes. *International Review for the Sociology of Sport, 43*(3), 227–249.

Haugen, K.K., & Popela, P. (2015). Why sports officials may choose not to fight performance-enhancing drugs. *European Journal of Sports Studies, 3*(2), 32–39.

Henne, K. (2014). The emergence of moral technopreneurialism in sport: Techniques in antidoping regulation, 1966–1976. *The International Journal of the History of Sport, 31*(8), 884–901.

Henning, A., & Dimeo, P. (2019). Perceptions of legitimacy, attitudes and buy-in among athlete groups: A cross-national qualitative investigation providing practical solutions. *The World Anti-Doping Agency.* Retrieved from https://www.wada-ama.org/en/resources/social-science/

Hong, F., (2006). Doping and anti-doping in sport in China: An analysis of recent and present attitudes and actions. *Sport in Society, 9,* 314–333. 10.1080/17430430500491348.

Houlihan, B. (2002a). *Dying to win: Doping in sport and the development of anti-doping policy* (Vol. 996). Strasbourg, France: Council of Europe Publishing.

Houlihan, B. (2002b). Managing compliance in international anti-doping policy: The World Anti-Doping Code. *European Sport Management Quarterly, 2*(3), 188–208.

Houlihan, Barrie (2009). Mechanisms of international influence on domestic elite sport policy. *International Journal of Sport Policy and Politics, 1,* 51–69. 10.1080/19406940 902739090.

Houlihan, B. (2014). Achieving compliance in international anti-doping policy: An analysis of the 2009 World Anti-Doping Code. *Sport Management Review, 17*(3), 265–276.

Houlihan, B., & Hanstad, D.V. (2019). The effectiveness of the World Anti-Doping Agency: Developing a framework for analysis. *International Journal of Sport Policy and Politics, 11*(2), 203–217.

Houlihan, B., & Preece, A. (2007). Independence and accountability: The case of the Drug Free Sport Directorate, the UK's national anti-doping organisation. *Public Policy and Administration, 22*(4), 381–402.

Hoye, R., Smith, A.C., Nicholson, M., & Stewart, B. (2015). *Sport management: Principles and applications.* Abingdon, UK: Routledge.

IOC. (2019). The Olympic Charter. Retrieved from https://stillmed.olympic.org/.

Jedlicka, S.R., & Hunt, T.M. (2013). The international anti-doping movement and UNESCO: A historical case study. *The International Journal of the History of Sport, 30*(13), 1523–1535.

Kamber, M. (2011). Development of the role of national anti-doping organisations in the fight against doping: From past to future. *Forensic Science International*, *213*(1–3), 3–9.

Kayser, B., & Smith, A.C. (2008). Globalisation of anti-doping: The reverse side of the medal. *British Medical Journal, 337*.

Kirby, K., Moran, A., & Guerin, S. (2011). A qualitative analysis of the experiences of elite athletes who have admitted to doping for performance enhancement. *International Journal of Sport Policy and Politics*, *3*(2), 205–224.

Krasner, S.D. Ed. (1983). *International regimes*. Ithaca, NY: Cornell University Press.

Kustec Lipicer, S., & McArdle, D. (2014). National law, domestic governance and global policy: A case study of anti-doping policy in Slovenia *International Journal of Sport Policy and Politics*, *6*(1), 71–87.

Maennig, W. (2014). Inefficiency of the anti-doping system: Cost reduction proposals. *Substance Use & Misuse*, *49*(9), 1201–1205.

Mazanov, J., & Connor, J. (2010). Rethinking the management of drugs in sport. *International Journal of Sport Policy*, *2*(1), 49–63.

Mahoney, D., (2018). Doping Appeals at the Court of Arbitration for Sport: Lessons from Essendon. *Boston College Law Review*, 59, 1807–1837.

Meyer, J.W., & Rowan, B. (1977). Institutionalized organizations: Formal structure as myth and ceremony. *American Journal of Sociology*, *83*(2), 340–363.

Moston, S., Engelberg, T., & Skinner, J. (2015). Athletes' and coaches' perceptions of deterrents to performance-enhancing drug use. *International Journal of Sport Policy and Politics*, 7, 623–636. 10.1080/19406940.2014.936960.

Møller, V. (2016). The road to hell is paved with good intentions—A critical evaluation of WADA's anti-doping campaign. *Performance Enhancement & Health*, *4*(3–4), 111–115.

Ohl, F., Fincoeur, B., Lentillon-Kaestner, V., Defrance, J., & Brissonneau, C. (2015). The socialization of young cyclists and the culture of doping. *International Review for the Sociology of Sport*, *50*(7), 865–882.

Overbye, M. (2016). Doping control in sport: An investigation of how elite athletes perceive and trust the functioning of the doping testing system in their sport. *Sport Management Review*, *19*(1), 6–22.

Overbye, M., & Wagner, U. (2014). Experiences, attitudes and trust: An inquiry into elite athletes' perception of the whereabouts reporting system. *International Journal of Sport Policy and Politics*, *6*(3), 407–428.

Overbye, M., Elbe, A.M., Knudsen, M.L., & Pfister, G. (2015). Athletes' perceptions of anti-doping sanctions: The ban from sport versus social, financial and self-imposed sanctions. *Sport in Society*, *18*(3), 364–384.

Overbye, M., Knudsen, M.L., & Pfister, G. (2013). To dope or not to dope: Elite athletes' perceptions of doping deterrents and incentives. *Performance Enhancement & Health*, *2*(3), 119–134.

Park, J.K. (2005). Governing doped bodies: The world anti-doping agency and the global culture of surveillance. *Cultural Studies ↔ Critical Methodologies*, *5*(2), 174–188.

Pound, R.W., Ayotte, C., Parkinson, A., Pengilly, A., & Ryan, A. (2013). *Report to WADA Executive Committee on lack of effectiveness of testing programs*. Canada: World Anti-Doping Agency.

Pratt, T.C., Cullen, F.T., Blevins, K.R., Daigle, L.E., & Madensen, T.D. (2006). The empirical status of deterrence theory: A meta-analysis. *Taking stock: The status of criminological theory* (pp. 367–396). New Jersey, NJ: Transaction Publishers.

Robinson, L. (2015). The business of sport. In B. Houlihan & D. Malcolm (Eds.), *Sport & society: A student introduction* (pp. 273–289). London: Sage.

Skille, E.Å., Hanstad, D.V., & Tjernsbekk, P.A. (2011). The institutionalization of national anti-doping work after the introduction of the World Anti-Doping Code. *International Journal of Applied Sports Sciences, 23*(2).

Skinner, J., Read, D., & Kihl, L.A. (2017). Applying a conceptual model of policy regime effectiveness to national and international anti-doping policy in sport. In *Corruption in Sport* (pp. 62–78). London, UK: Routledge.

Strelan, P., & Boeckmann, R.J. (2006). Why drug testing in elite sport does not work: Perceptual deterrence theory and the role of personal moral beliefs. *Journal of Applied Social Psychology, 36*(12), 2909–2934.

Suchman, M.C. (1995). Managing legitimacy: Strategic and institutional approaches. *Academy of Management Review, 20*(3), 571–610.

Tamburrini, C. (2006). Are doping sanctions justified? A moral relativistic view. *Sport in Society, 9*(2), 199–211.

Tan, T.C., Bairner, A., & Chen, Y.W. (2020). Managing compliance with the World Anti-Doping Code: China's strategies and their implications. *International Review for the Sociology of Sport, 55*(3), 251–271.

Thompson, A., & Verdier, D. (2014). Multilateralism, bilateralism, and regime design. *International Studies Quarterly, 58*(1), 15–28.

Toohey, K., & Beaton, A. (2017). International cross-sector social partnerships between sport and governments: The World Anti-Doping Agency. *Sport Management Review, 20*(5), 483–496.

Ulrich, R., Pope, H.G., Cléret, L., Petróczi, A., Nepusz, T., Schaffer, J., & Simon, P. (2018). Doping in two elite athletics competitions assessed by randomized-response surveys. *Sports Medicine, 48*(1), 211–219.

WADA. (2019). Compliance strategy. World Anti-Doping Agency. Retrieved from https://www.wada-ama.org/sites/default/files/20200326_compliance_strategy.pdf.

WADA. (2020a). 135th IOC session. Lausanne: 10 January 2020. Speech by Witold Banka, WADA president. World Anti-Doping Agency. Retrieved from https://www.wada-ama.org/sites/default/files/resources/files/20200110_extraordinaryiocsession_wb.pdf

WADA. (2020b). Who We Are. World Anti-Doping Agency. Retrieved from https://www.wada-ama.org/en/who-we-are.

WADA. (2020c). WADA's regional offices – Protecting clean sport around the world. World Anti-Doping Agency. Retrieved from https://www.wada-ama.org/en/media/news/2020-05/wadas-regional-offices-protecting-clean-sport-around-the-world.

Waddington, I., & Møller, V. (2019). WADA at twenty: Old problems and old thinking? *International Journal of Sport Policy and Politics, 11*(2), 219–231.

Wagner, U. (2009). The World Anti-Doping Agency: Constructing a hybrid organisation in permanent stress (dis)order? *International Journal of Sport Policy, 1*(2), 183–201.

Wagner, U. (2010). The International Cycling Union under Siege—Anti-doping and the Biological Passport as a Mission Impossible? *European Sport Management Quarterly, 10*, 321–342. 10.1080/16184741003770206.

Wagner, U., & Hanstad, D. V. (2011). Scandinavian perspectives on doping – a comparative policy analysis in relation to the international process of institutionalizing anti-doping. *International Journal of Sport Policy and Politics, 3*, 355–372. 10.1080/19406940.2011.596156.

Wenn, S., Barney, R., & Martyn, S. (2011). *Tarnished rings: The international Olympic committee and the Salt Lake City bid scandal.* Syracuse, NY: Syracuse University Press.

Westmattelmann, D., Dreiskämper, D., Strauß, B., Schewe, G., & Plass, J. (2018). Perception of the current anti-doping regime – A quantitative study among German top-level cyclists and track and field athletes. *Frontiers in Psychology*, 9, 1890.

Woolway, T., Lazuras, L., Barkoukis, V., & Petróczi, A. (2020). 'Doing what is right and doing it right': A mapping review of athletes' perception of anti-doping legitimacy. *International Journal of Drug Policy*, 84.

Zucker, L. G. (1977). The role of institutionalization in cultural persistence. *American Sociological Review*, 42(5), 726–743.

Chapter 2

Multi-level legitimacy

We started this book by highlighting that anti-doping efforts are undermined by the exposure of socially organised doping scandals. Despite World Anti-Doping Agency's (WADA) efforts and successes over the past 20 years, organisations and nations have been able to engage in large-scale doping practices. Having established that WADA's progress towards its goal of doping-free sport has been challenged by a lack of behavioural support from signatories, there is a utility in using theories of organisational behaviour to study *why* this has occurred. Institutional theorists (Meyer & Rowan, 1977; Zucker, 1977) view organisational behaviour as a combination of rational decision-making and social pressures. It rests on three related concepts: institutions, the field and legitimacy to explain organisational behaviour.

Firstly, institutional theory provides a framework in which 'institutions' act as cultural pressures that infer modes of normal (or accepted) behaviour. In anti-doping, the use of performance-enhancing drug (PED) is one behaviour that violates institutional norms. Secondly, a field is a group of related organisations that interact around a shared issue (e.g., WADA, the International Olympic Committee (IOC) and national governments). Finally, the term *legitimacy* denotes the perceived appropriateness of an organisation's behaviour in relation to social expectations within a field (Deephouse, Bundy, Tost, & Suchman, 2017). Taken together, these three concepts make sense of why different organisations behave in similar ways. That is, once organisations, products, services, techniques, policies, programs or beliefs become institutionalised, members of the field adopt them to appear legitimate – even if they do not directly improve technical performance (DiMaggio & Powell, 1983; Jepperson, 1991; Meyer & Rowan, 1977). WADA can be understood as an institution that places institutional pressures on members of the field of anti-doping to conform with the policies and programs set out in the World Anti-Doping Code (WADC) (Wagner, 2010).

A cursory examination of the history of WADA indicates that signatories have not always abided by the WADC. It is possible for individuals and organisations to resist institutional pressures and challenge the legitimacy of an institution (Oliver, 1991; Pache & Santos, 2010). The identified lack of behavioural support for WADA can be understood as a form of stakeholder resistance against institutional pressures to conform with the WADC. This creates a dynamic multi-level relationship between (1) the legitimacy of an institution that is the source of the normative pressures applied to actors in a field and (2) organisations in a field that are subject to institutional pressures. We aim to analyse the legitimacy of WADA in relation to how it has been challenged and how it has responded. In doing so, insight into the reasons why WADA has experienced a lack of support can be identified.

Accordingly, this chapter introduces the construct of multi-level legitimacy and its value as an analytical tool to understand and explain the challenges WADA confronts. We begin this discussion by introducing institutional theory and organisational legitimacy. Secondly, we outline multi-level legitimacy theory (Bitektine & Haack, 2015) to structure the analysis of how the legitimacy of WADA has been challenged and how the organisation has responded. This is supported by discussion of previous research which has addressed the legitimacy of WADA to demonstrate the multi-level nature of legitimacy specific to the organisation. Finally, we conclude by explaining how the case studies selected to study WADA's legitimacy were chosen and the sources of data used in the analysis.

What is an institution?

Institutions are features of fields that prescribe appropriate modes of behaviour (i.e., 'institutional pressures'). Building on this, an institution can be either structural (e.g., an organisation such as WADA) or cultural (e.g., marriage; Jepperson, 1991). The WADA regime prescribes how athletes and sporting organisations should behave. Definitions of the term 'institutions' vary and have divided organisational scholars (Scott, 2008). Greenwood, Oliver, Suddaby, and Sahlin-Andersson (2008) defined an institution as 'a more-or-less taken-for-granted repetitive social behaviour that is underpinned by normative systems and cognitive understandings that give meaning to social exchange and thus enable self-reproducing social order' (p. 4–5). Similarly, Scott (2008) defined the term as 'social structures that have attained a high degree of resilience and are composed of cultural-cognitive, normative, and regulative elements that, together with associated activities and resources, provide stability and meaning to social life'. These definitions, although not comprehensive, described institutions as sets of social expectations that are somewhat resistant to change. WADA, as an organisation, satisfies these criteria as it creates clear institutional pressures on anti-doping field members. We are not the first to treat the WADA regime as an institution. Wagner (2010) stated:

> Anti-doping measures can be defined as an institution. Testing regimes, surveillance structures, legal bodies, the listing of prohibited substances, educational programmes and scientific research are all examples of the ongoing international process of institutionalizing anti-doping measures in

sport ... since 1999, the closer contact between sports federations and governments and the pressure on sports organisations to comply with the common set of rules (the WADC) have accelerated the process. (p. 332)

From an institutional perspective, the WADA regime prescribes appropriate behaviour for individuals and groups (institutional pressures) that constitute the field of anti-doping (Hanstad & Houlihan, 2015; Skille, Hanstad, & Tjernsbekk, 2011).

Early work on institutional theory positioned isomorphic processes as key factors leading to similarities between organisations in a field (DiMaggio & Powell, 1983; Meyer & Rowan, 1977). Isomorphism is the idea that organisations in a field begin to resemble each other because of conformity to institutional pressures. In the field of anti-doping, national governments created national anti-doping organisations (NADOs) responsible for managing testing of that nation's athletes would be an example of an institutional pressure created by WADA that has led to isomorphism. Institutional pressures can be differentiated into mimetic, coercive and normative pressures. Mimetic pressures occur because certain characteristics of successful organisations are viewed as necessary for success. Coercive pressures exist due to obligatory regulatory standards (e.g., adoption of health and safety protocols). Normative pressures occur because clients and other stakeholders come to expect certain characteristics associated with a profession or industry.

Arguments about isomorphism and institutional theory suffer from a limitation because neither explains how institutions change. Organisations are treated as passive agents that are subject to institutional pressures with no capacity to challenge existing institutions or create new ones. Clearly, to make sense of WADA's legitimacy, this premise is insufficient to explain the disagreements that exist in relation to anti-doping policy and practice. The field of anti-doping and the existence of WADA have been characterised by different stakeholders seeking to challenge its legitimacy (Read, Skinner, Lock, & Houlihan, 2019). Therefore, we require a framework that explains why stakeholders actively resist or challenge institutional pressures. As we will argue, institutional change can be explained by appreciating that fields contain a diverse array of actors that possess different judgements about the legitimacy of an institution.

Legitimacy, institutional complexity and change

Early theorists proposed that legitimacy was bestowed upon organisations that complied with an institution and institutional pressures (i.e., isomorphism). In turn, compliance led to support, resources and organisational survival (Hamilton, 2006; Zimmerman & Zeitz, 2002). The argument that organisations in a field appear to mimic one another in the pursuit of legitimacy is supported by evidence that organisations copy successful practices and behaviours (e.g., Deephouse, 1996, 1999; Glynn & Abzug, 2002; Heugens & Lander, 2009;

Staw & Epstein, 2000; Wu & Salomon, 2016). Understanding isomorphism becomes more complex when considering that organisations may exist in a field characterised by multiple ideas (i.e., logics) or operate in multiple fields each with different normative pressures (Kostova & Zaheer, 1999; Raynard, 2016).

Groups of institutions and institutional pressures within a field form socially structured orders of practice, termed *institutional logics* (Friedland & Alford, 1991). Institutional logics are defined as 'the socially constructed, historical patterns of material practices, assumptions, values, beliefs, and rules by which individuals produce and reproduce their material subsistence, organize time and space, and provide meaning to their social reality' (Thornton & Ocasio, 1999, p. 804). For example, in the field of Olympic sport there are multiple simultaneous logics (e.g., commercialism and nationalism) that place institutional pressures on field members to behave in certain ways. Multiple institutional pressures can be compatible and unproblematic, a state referred to as *institutional pluralism* (Kraatz & Block, 2008). Equally, multiple institutional pressures can be conflicting, which is labelled as *institutional complexity* (Greenwood, Raynard, Kodeih, Micelotta, & Lounsbury, 2011). Under conditions of institutional complexity, organisations are required to navigate different pressures using strategic responses that vary in the degree to which each is accepted or supported. Organisational responses to institutional pressures and legitimacy challenges can be broadly categorised along a continuum of resistance, from full acquiescence to compromise, avoidance, defiance and manipulation (Oliver, 1991). Combinations of different responses can lead to new organisational structures and policies, or the separation and prioritisation of expectations from different stakeholders (e.g., Boxenbaum & Jonsson, 2008; Bromley & Powell, 2012; MacLean & Behnam, 2010; Pache & Santos, 2010, 2013; Westphal & Zajac, 2001). The presence of different organisational responses to competing logics indicates that organisations have agency to deal with institutional pressures (Ashforth & Gibbs, 1990; Baron, Dobbin, & Jennings, 1986). This is evident in the field of anti-doping as the International Association of Athletics Federations (IAAF), which rebranded itself as World Athletics in 2019, and the International Federation of Association Football (FIFA) took different approaches to the institutional pressures emerging from the introduction of WADA (Wagner, 2011). World Athletics proactively engaged with WADA whilst FIFA displayed greater scepticism towards the new organisation. Ultimately, the capacity for organisations to resist institutional pressures also enables the possibility to challenge the legitimacy of an institution, which may lead to institutional change.

Recently there has been a shift in research emphasis from understanding why organisations resemble one another to explaining how individuals and organisations respond to institutional pressures (Alvesson & Spicer, 2019). Although institutions are features of social life, they change as a result of how individuals communicate and interpret institutional pressures (Powell & Colyvas, 2008). Furthermore, if we are to understand how institutions change, there is a need to understand how individuals that resist institutional pressures contribute to the process. The difficulty in explaining change in institutions, such as WADA, through micro-level behaviours of individuals is the paradox of embedded agency (Battilana, Leca, & Boxenbaum, 2009; Holm, 1995; Seo & Creed, 2002). The embedded agency paradox poses: 'How can actors change institutions if their actions, intentions, and rationality are all conditioned by the very institution they wish to change?' (Holm, 1995, p. 398). This paradox implies that WADA's legitimacy could not be challenged because stakeholders and organisations within the field of anti-doping have been conditioned by institutional pressures. However, the organisational history of WADA indicates that its legitimacy has been frequently resisted and challenged by stakeholders in the field of anti-doping (Dimeo & Møller, 2018; Read et al., 2019). Therefore, in addressing the embedded agency paradox we critically analyse how the legitimacy of WADA has been challenged, and how WADA has responded. As we will argue in the next section, by conceptualising legitimacy as a judgement rendered by individual evaluators about an organisation (Suddaby, Bitektine, & Haack, 2017) we can achieve two conceptual outcomes. Firstly, we can use institutional theory to explain how WADA creates institutional pressures that shape individual and organisational behaviour in the field of anti-doping. Secondly, by incorporating multi-level legitimacy theorising, we can make sense of how the actions of individuals and organisations within the field of anti-doping have led to institutional change.

Multi-level legitimacy theory

Treating legitimacy as an individual-level perception (Suddaby et al., 2017) invokes a position from which an organisation's legitimacy, and hence the behavioural support it garners, can be determined by how evaluators (e.g., individuals, organisations, the media, the state) judge it against pragmatic, moral and cognitive criteria (Deephouse et al., 2017; Suchman, 1995). This is reflected in Deephouse et al's. (2017) definition of legitimacy: 'Legitimacy is the perceived appropriateness of an organization to a social system in terms of rules, values, norms, and definitions' (p. 32). In this section we introduce multi-level legitimacy theory and explain three key concepts pivotal to understanding the multi-level legitimacy of WADA: (1) judgement of propriety, (2) consensus and (3) validity.

Judgement of propriety

Multi-level legitimacy theory (Bitektine & Haack, 2015) is a process model that connects individuals and institutions to explain the stability of an institution's legitimacy. The theory is predominantly based on the work of Bitektine (2011) who proposed that individual evaluators can actively judge or passively accept the legitimacy of an organisation. It also relied heavily on the work of Tost (2011) who distinguished the two related concepts of propriety judgements and validity.

Individual evaluators judge the degree to which organisational actions are proper (i.e., propriety) or appropriate (Haack, Schilke, & Zucker, 2020; Lock, Filo, Kunkel, & Skinner, 2015; Weber, 1978). These judgements can be influenced by personal benefits derived from the institution (pragmatic criteria), societal benefits derived from the institution (moral criteria), and their ability to comprehend the purpose of the institution (cognitive criteria). In the case of WADA, individual evaluators in the field of anti-doping, such as NADOs, will judge the propriety of WADA based on what the organisation offers to them, the anti-doping field and what they perceive as the purpose of WADA.

Athlete perceptions provide a good example of propriety judgements about WADA. Researchers have addressed athlete perceptions of WADC policy implementation, concluding that athletes perceived current anti-doping rules as legitimate due to necessity, but implementation as illegitimate due to inconsistencies between NADOs (e.g., Bloodworth & McNamee, 2010; Efverström, Ahmadi, Hoff, & Bäckström, 2016; Henning & Dimeo, 2019; Overbye & Wagner, 2014). A systematic review of previous research examining how athletes perceived the legitimacy of anti-doping organisations and testing supported that legitimacy judgements are multi-faceted (Woolway, Lazuras, Barkoukis, & Petróczi, 2020). Based on a sample of 13,487 athletes from 39 identified studies, Woolway et al. argued that anti-doping was typically perceived as the right thing to do to protect sport by those surveyed, but there were negative judgements of the propriety of anti-doping policies and procedures to achieve this objective. Woolway et al. suggested this may undermine compliance with the WADC by athletes.

Consensus and validity

Validity refers to institutionalised perceptions of organisational appropriateness at a collective macro-level (Dornbush & Scott, 1975). The collective may be an organisation, a social group or an entire field. Within this collective, there will be a judgement of legitimacy (i.e., legitimate or illegitimate) which individual evaluators perceive to be dominant. The dominant or 'valid' judgement in a field will be determined by propriety judgements expressed by important field members such as the media, government and regulatory bodies in the form of validity cues. As a result, validity cues shape understanding about expected behaviours in a field. Individual evaluators then passively accept an organisation until given reason to actively evaluate it or look for further cues about its validity (Bitektine & Haack, 2015). For an institution such as WADA, there will be a diverse array of judgements about the organisation's propriety at an individual micro-level. However, there will be a single dominant collective perception of legitimacy (i.e., validity) that determines institutional pressures and represents the macro-level phenomenon of legitimacy. We argue that WADA is legitimate because it exerts institutional pressures on members of the field of anti-doping to behave according to the WADC.

Importantly to our discussion of WADA's legitimacy, a dominant collective validity judgement does not imply that there is consensus between individual evaluators about the legitimacy of an institution (Haack et al., 2020). It is possible for an individual to privately maintain a negative judgement about the legitimacy of an institution that he or she may conceal if he or she perceives that other individuals in the field oppose his or her view. As such, there may be disagreement between field members about the legitimacy of an institution. The extent of this disagreement can range from high to low consensus (Haack et al., 2020). When there is high consensus (i.e., strong validity), there is minimal disagreement about the propriety of an organisation, and validity is largely a coalescence of positive evaluations. Under conditions of low consensus (i.e., weak validity), the macro-level legitimacy of an institution does not reflect the various judgements of propriety held by individual evaluators and is, therefore, an 'illusion of support' (Haack et al., 2020). As we will argue, WADA's legitimacy at a macro-level is inherently vulnerable due to a lack of consensus between judgements of propriety.

The field of anti-doping is characterised by multiple judgements of WADA's legitimacy. Houlihan (2009) suggested that countries and sport organisations may engage with anti-doping policy as the discourse around the issue has gained powerful public and media support. Through campaigning, WADA has promoted anti-doping to increase its perceived legitimacy (Qvarfordt Hoff, Bäckström, & Ahmadi, 2019; Toohey & Beaton, 2017; Wagner, 2011). Anti-doping is now at a point where, because of institutional pressures, sport organisations must at least appear to be concerned about doping, even if they do not privately value it. Girginov (2006) proposed that agreeing to the WADC may be a result of isomorphic pressures, citing the Bulgarian Weightlifting Federation's attempts to be concerned with anti-doping. Similarly, following the Lahti doping scandal in which six Finnish cross-country skiers were found to have committed anti-doping violations, the International Skiing Federation adopted the WADC in 2001 to demonstrate its commitment to anti-doping efforts (Hanstad, 2008). Wagner (2010, 2011) argued that as the issue of drugs in sport and WADA have become the prevailing judgement in the field of anti-doping, the isomorphic pressures acting on sport organisations to comply with the WADC have increased as they strive to maintain their own legitimacy. He also noted that sports organisations have utilised strategies to mitigate the threat of anti-doping to commercial objectives, thus undermining WADA's legitimacy. These findings portray a situation where, despite the apparent in-stitutionalisation of anti-doping as an important issue in sport, variability in judgements about the propriety of anti-doping can undermine the legitimacy of WADA and in turn the WADC.

Stability and suppressor factors

The multi-level legitimacy model (Bitektine & Haack, 2015) emphasises the conditions under which deviant judgements of propriety are expressed or suppressed. Under conditions of institutional stability, there is a prevailing collective judgement of legitimacy (i.e., validity). Institutional stability is maintained by suppressor factors. Suppressor factors are what an individual perceives as the positive or negative repercussions for expressing a propriety judgement that contrasts or challenges dominant institutions. Suppressor factors rely on individuals believing (correctly or not) that there will be negative consequences for disagreeing with the dominant judgement, such as threat of legal action, social disapproval or reputational concerns. Consequently, individuals will comply with institutional pressures (at least superficially). In the field of anti-doping, for example, signatories to the WADC may judge WADA as illegitimate but suppress this perception and comply superficially with the WADC to avoid the negative repercussions.

By appreciating that an institution can be collectively perceived as legitimate despite contrasting judgements of propriety that are suppressed by institutional pressures, we are able to explain the paradox of embedded agency. We develop this argument in the next section to explain how institutional change can occur and how the level of consensus can be examined.

Jolts and conditions for change

Institutions and fields are dynamic, and open to change. Judgements of propriety and suppressor factors can be used to explain how change may occur. In a period of institutional stability, deviant propriety judgements are suppressed. However, events can initiate reconsideration about the legitimacy of an institution and pave the way for institutional change. Such events act as jolts, which provide new information about institutions. In turn, the exposure of new information provides individual evaluators with content to update or change judgements of organisational propriety. For example, the exposure of the Russian Olympic doping scandal revealed new information to members of the anti-doping field that the current testing protocols could be subverted. Stakeholders then used this cue to re-evaluate the appropriateness of WADA's behaviour.

Jolts can create conditions for institutional change. When institutional stability is reduced, previously suppressed judgements can be expressed to challenge the collective validity with reduced fear of repercussions. Jolts may also cause other individual evaluators to reconsider the legitimacy of an institution, especially if the deviant propriety judgement comes from an important source (e.g., the government or legal system). In the example of the Russian Olympic doping scandal, WADA's legitimacy was debated as a host of different organisations and individuals challenged WADA's behaviour. In the ensuing debate, WADA responded to the challenges by changing structures and processes to address concerns demonstrating how change can occur after jolts.

In addition to understanding how jolts lead to institutional change, it is also critical to examine the period of legitimacy debate following contextual changes. Doing so provides an opportunity to investigate the level of consensus between different judgements about the propriety of anti-doping and WADA. As individuals and organisations take advantage of the reduced suppressor factors to express deviant judgements in order to challenge WADA's legitimacy, it is possible to analyse on what criteria WADA's legitimacy is evaluated. It also provides an opportunity to study how WADA has handled challenges to its legitimacy. For example, athletes may render a legitimacy judgement of WADA based on moral criteria that they expect the organisation to protect the athlete community. Equally, International Federations may render a judgement about how well WADA protects its own needs, potentially creating contradictory behavioural expectations. How WADA manages varying expectations of legitimate behaviour and the approach it chooses will have wide-ranging consequences.

There is limited work that has directly attended to WADA's attempts to manage its legitimacy as a regulatory body. McDermott, Henne, and Connor (2013) considered the relationship between cultural beliefs about doping in sport and the perceived legitimacy of WADA's mission. They proposed that the perceived legitimacy of WADA, and hence compliance with the WADC, would be greater if WADA considered that evaluations of legitimacy are related to culture and context. Gowthorp, Greenhow, and O'Brien (2016) supported this argument, finding that legitimacy derived from being in a position of authority is insufficient to successfully conduct anti-doping activities. Anti-doping organisations also need to be perceived as legitimate to achieve support. McDermott (2015) linked legitimacy with moral panics. Moral panics are events that are portrayed so that they appear to threaten social values so that an organisation can justify controlling the situation. She noted that the presence and exposure of doping constitutes a legitimacy crisis for governing organisations such as the IOC, and in order to restore perceptions of legitimacy, doping is portrayed as a moral panic that allows these organisations to take control of the situation.

The implication for WADA's legitimacy as the chief regulator of anti-doping is that it must demonstrate independence from the IOC. In an attempt to display independence, and to enhance legitimacy, in 2002, WADA was based in Montreal, Canada (Toohey & Beaton, 2017). Equally, when WADA has exercised its independence as a regulatory agency and challenged the IOC, it was perceived to be overstepping its responsibilities (Read et al., 2019). Finally, analysis of WADA guides explaining the WADC provided to athletes suggested that the organisation has progressively sought to legitimate its activities with athlete-centred arguments rather than authoritarian reasoning (Qvarfordt et al., 2019). Evidently, WADA's active attempts to manage its legitimacy as a regulatory body have presented in different forms, with differing levels of success.

We have argued that periods of institutional change and legitimacy debates that follow jolts provide an excellent opportunity to assess the level of consensus within the field of anti-doping as members express judgements of propriety about WADA. By understanding the consensus underpinning the validity of WADA's legitimacy, it is possible to understand the stability of the organisation and reasons for a lack of behavioural support. Further, WADA has the capacity to actively manage its legitimacy. The final section of this chapter will explain how the case studies used to explore WADA's legitimacy were chosen and how data was obtained to analyse the legitimacy processes.

Case study selection

We use multiple case studies to examine the legitimacy processes around the WADA regime. In this section we outline how the seven cases were chosen. Merriam (1998) states that case studies focus on insights rather than hypothesis testing, defining a case study as 'an intensive, holistic description and analysis of a bounded phenomenon such as a program, an institution, a person, a process, or a social unit' (p. xiii). The bounded system, also known as the unit of analysis, is a clear object (e.g., person, organisation, policy) of a phenomenon (e.g., social change, innovation, deviance). For example, the object in this book is the WADA regime, and the phenomenon is the processes of institutional change and stability proposed by multi-level legitimacy (Bitektine & Haack, 2015).

In order to be selected for analysis, cases needed to be information-rich demonstrating multi-level legitimacy processes relevant to the construction of WADA's legitimacy. To identify appropriate cases, we conducted a search using Nexis.com. Nexis.com is a database and search engine with global coverage for media outlets. A keyword search was conducted for any articles containing 'World Anti-Doping Agency' once and 'WADA' at least three times. This search spanned from the creation of WADA in 1999 to June 2020 and included all newspaper articles published globally in English. The rationale for the word search is that media coverage was used to assess the extent to which the WADA regime, and by proxy, its legitimacy, was discussed both positively and negatively after jolts and/or challenges. These articles were screened to identify potential cases that would provide information-rich examples. The purpose of the screening was twofold. Firstly, to find cases in which the legitimacy of WADA had been challenged, and secondly, to identify issues that led to WADA publicly responding to manage its legitimacy. We compiled a list of issues in six-month blocks (e.g., July 2000–December 2000) that caused WADA to be discussed in the media since its creation (see Appendix A). From this list, we identified case studies, excluded duplicates and limited only to publications in English.

The decision was made to include a case study focused on the legitimacy processes at the Lausanne Conference, which led to the creation of WADA. The rationale for this decision was to investigate how institutional change at Lausanne suppressed and validated different legitimacy judgements within the organisational field. Underpinning the multi-level legitimacy theory is the assumption that there are suppressed individuals and organisations in the field of anti-doping and that following jolts deviant judgements are expressed. Given this, we believe there is a need to understand how the creation of WADA suppressed evaluator's propriety judgements and how this suppression facilitated subsequent legitimacy challenges.

The case selection criteria were based on the focus and volume of content. Stories that did not lead to challenges directly to WADA were excluded (e.g., athlete anti-doping rule violations), as were stories that generated only a small amount of press coverage (less than five articles) and story coverage that was deemed to be to geographically focused. For these reasons, there are three event case studies and three policy case studies that are relevant to our analysis of the WADA regime. Event case studies are specific scandals that challenged the legitimacy of WADA. The event case studies focus on the Lance Armstrong, Essendon Australian Football League club and Russian Olympic doping scandals. These events generated significant press coverage and scrutiny over an extended amount of time, providing a large dataset. Policy case studies include situations in which anti-doping rules have led to WADA's legitimacy being debated. The policy case studies include the athlete whereabouts system, therapeutic use exemptions (TUE) and the prohibition of recreational drugs. Within each of these policies were stories about athletes that did not individually create a large amount of press coverage or were geographically centralised, but the policy in general has consistently led to WADA's legitimacy being challenged. These policy cases reflect broader narratives about the legitimacy of WADA (e.g., British athlete Christine Ohuruogu's whereabouts system violation) and improve the geographic coverage of stories that might have been excluded on their own (e.g., the Board of Control for Cricket in India questioning the whereabouts system).

Data collection

To explore the legitimacy of WADA two sources of data were used in the case studies: newspaper reports and WADA organisational documents.

Newspaper reports

News reports are becoming an increasingly valuable data source in sport policy and anti-doping research (e.g., Broch & Skille, 2019; Ritchie & Jackson, 2014; Heinze & Lu, 2017; Starke & Flemming, 2017). Brundage (2017) states that the quotes and statements of individuals presented in newspaper articles can provide a source of primary data. These statements are recorded at the time of communication for the purpose of public communication. Therefore, quotes presented in a newspaper article can be used to support the analysis of WADA's legitimacy. Accordingly, for each case study, Nexis.com was used to identify relevant articles. The specific search protocols (e.g., search terms, dates, number of articles) for each case are presented in each chapter. News reports help identify how [and which] individual evaluators challenged the legitimacy of WADA after jolts and how WADA responded. From newspaper data alone, it is not possible to determine the inner working of an organisation, and caution must be exercised when discussing why an organisation may have made a particular argument or point. However, this is not considered problematic as this book is concerned with the public expression, debate and construction of judgements in relation to WADA's legitimacy as well as the organisation's strategic responses.

Other benefits of newspaper reports as a form of data include the ability to analyse different points of view within the same article and that they act as a form of snowball sampling by signposting other relevant sources of information (e.g., press releases). Further, the retrospective view means that the individual evaluators who shaped the dominant legitimacy judgement in relation to an issue can be identified alongside the individuals and organisations who were eventually suppressed. Finally, the media and journalists have the potential to influence the judgements of their readerships and constitute a source of legitimacy (Walsh & McAllister-Spooner, 2011). Therefore, in addition to the quotes and statements that articles provide, journalists play a major role in legitimacy processes as a validity cue to other individual evaluators of what is and is not acceptable (Bitektine & Haack, 2015).

We acknowledge that the bias of the writer, the editing process and the newspaper need to be considered when relying upon newspaper articles as a source of primary data. Therefore, newspaper articles should not be limited to major publishers for availability. Nexis is a repository and search engine for newspaper articles published globally. The use of Nexis reduced the selection bias (i.e., selecting newspaper outlets a priori) and distance bias (i.e., only using newspaper outlets geographically close to the event) inherent in relying upon purposefully sampled newspaper outlets (Ortiz, Myers, Walls, & Diaz, 2005). As a result, our samples consist of a diverse array of articles from publishers globally. Articles shorter than 500 words and website sources, magazines, industry trade press and blogs were deleted to remove duplicates from newspaper websites and remove user-generated content to improve validity (Henning & Dimeo, 2015).

WADA organisational documents

Naturally occurring documents (i.e., without researcher initiation) have the potential benefit of being less prone to response bias and editorialising. Organisational documents included press releases, the WADC, WADA Executive Committee meetings minutes, WADA Foundation Board meetings' minutes and annual reports. The purpose of analysing naturally occurring documents is to provide insights about how organisations have challenged WADA and how WADA has responded to scrutiny. WADA attempts to construct how its legitimacy is perceived through these documents (Silverman, 2015; Qvarfordt et al., 2019). The remainder of this section will outline the different documentary sources we have drawn upon.

The first document source was press releases. Press releases provide direct commentary from an organisation about its judgements and intentions.

Although the genuineness of beliefs, motivations and behaviours presented in a press release or public statement can be contested by other individual evaluators, such releases constitute an important part of the institutional processes surrounding WADA's legitimacy.

The second document source is the WADC, which is a living document that is updated every four years in consultation with WADA's stakeholders. The purpose of the WADC is to detail the policies applicable to all stakeholders for harmonising anti-doping practice between sports and nations. The code is subject to continual revisions so that WADA and other stakeholders have the necessary powers and tactics to face the changing demands of anti-doping. Consequently, identifying and examining the historical changes in the WADC offer insight into the powers WADA thought was necessary to remain legitimate in the fight against anti-doping.

The third source of documents were provided by the WADA Executive Committee meeting minutes. The purpose of minutes is to record issues discussed, queries raised and decisions made. The Executive Committee meeting minutes provide an insight into the issues that challenged WADA's leaders, the responses discussed and the perceived advantages and disadvantages of each strategy. WADA Executive Committee meeting minutes consequently revealed aspects of how the organisation's legitimacy was challenged and how these challenges were confronted. Analysis of the minutes also sheds light on the priorities of the committee, what it perceived to be WADA's legitimate purpose and what it perceived was expected of WADA.

The final source was WADA's annual report documents, which contain a message from the president and director general and detail WADA's activities over the previous 12 months. They also reflect on the troubles experienced and any changes in strategy for the future. Linsley and Kajuter (2008) recommend that annual reports can be used by organisations to legitimate themselves by communicating strategies to stakeholders and identify strategic trends. Therefore, through WADA's annual reports, we argue that changes in strategies can be identified over the lifespan of the organisation.

Conclusion

In this chapter we have introduced institutional theory as a framework to examine organisational behaviour. Institutions are social structures that generate institutional pressures that guide legitimate and appropriate behaviour in an institutional field. In this sense, we argue that WADA is a structural institution in the field of anti-doping that pressures stakeholders to conform with the expectations set out in the WADC. Multi-level legitimacy theory develops the relationship between institutions, field and legitimacy to suggest that (1) there may be a lack of consensus about the legitimacy of an institution, and (2) following major events and jolts, field members are able to debate the legitimacy of an institution. Therefore, legitimacy is a two-way process, as an institution creates institutional pressures of legitimate behaviour in periods of stability; however, during periods of change, field members can debate the legitimacy of an institution. This requires that an examination of WADA's legitimacy and behavioural support considers how WADA's legitimacy has been challenged and how WADA responded. In the chapters that follow we present seven case studies that examine the legitimacy of WADA. We begin this analysis by examining the legitimacy processes that were employed at the Lausanne Conference that led to the creation of WADA.

References

Alvesson, M., & Spicer, A. (2019). Neo-institutional theory and organization studies: A mid-life crisis? *Organization Studies, 40*(2), 199–218.

Ashforth, B.E., & Gibbs, B.W. (1990). The double-edge of organizational legitimation. *Organization Science, 1*(2), 177–194.

Baron, J.N., Dobbin, F.R., & Jennings, P.D. (1986). War and peace: The evolution of modern personnel administration in US industry. *American Journal of Sociology, 92*(2), 350–383.

Battilana, J., Leca, B., & Boxenbaum, E. (2009). How actors change institutions: Towards a theory of institutional entrepreneurship. *Academy of Management Annals, 3*(1), 65–107.

Bitektine, A. (2011). Toward a theory of social judgments of organizations: The case of legitimacy, reputation, and status. *Academy of Management Review, 36*(1), 151–179.

Bitektine, A., & Haack, P. (2015). The 'macro' and the 'micro' of legitimacy: Toward a multilevel theory of the legitimacy process. *Academy of Management Review, 40*(1), 49–75.

Bloodworth, A., & McNamee, M. (2010). Clean Olympians? Doping and anti-doping: The views of talented young British athletes. *International Journal of Drug Policy, 21*(4), 276–282.

Boxenbaum, E., & Jonsson, S. (2008). Isomorphism, diffusion and decoupling. In R. Greenwood, C. Oliver, T. Lawrence, & R.E. Meyer (Eds.), *The Sage Handbook of Organizational Institutionalism* (pp. 78–98). Thousand Oaks, CA: Sage.

Broch, T. B., & Skille, E. Å. (2019). Performing sport political legitimacy: A cultural sociology perspective on sport politics. *Sociology of Sport Journal, 36*, 171–178. 10.1123/ssj.2017-0204.

Bromley, P., & Powell, W.W. (2012). From smoke and mirrors to walking the talk: Decoupling in the contemporary world. *Academy of Management Annals, 6*(1), 483–530.

Brundage, A. (2017). Going to the sources: A guide to historical research and writing, London, UK: John Wiley & Sons.

Deephouse, D.L. (1996). Does isomorphism legitimate? *Academy of Management Journal, 39*(4), 1024–1039.

Deephouse, D.L. (1999). To be different, or to be the same? It's a question (and theory) of strategic balance. *Strategic Management Journal, 20*(2), 147–166.

Deephouse, D.L., Bundy, J., Tost, L.P., & Suchman, M.C. (2017). Organizational legitimacy: Six key questions. In R. Greenwood et al. (Eds.), *The Sage handbook of organizational institutionalism* (2nd ed.). Thousand Oaks, CA: Sage.

DiMaggio, P., & Powell, W.W. (1983). The iron cage revisited: Collective rationality and institutional isomorphism in organizational fields. *American Sociological Review*, 48(2), 147–160.

Dimeo, P., & Møller, V. (2018). The anti-doping crisis in sport: Causes, consequences, solutions. London, UK: Routledge.

Dornbush, S.M., & Scott, W.R. (1975). *Evaluation and the exercise of authority*. San Francisco, CA: JosseyBass.

Efverström, A., Ahmadi, N., Hoff, D., & Bäckström, Å. (2016). Anti-doping and legitimacy: An international survey of elite athletes' perceptions. *International Journal of Sport Policy and Politics*, 8(3), 491–514.

Friedland, R., & Alford, R.R. (1991). Bringing society back in: Symbols, practices and institutional contradictions. In W.W. Powell & P.J. DiMaggio (Eds.), *The new institutionalism in organizational analysis* (pp. 232–267). Chicago, IL: University of Chicago Press.

Girginov, V. (2006). Creating a corporate anti-doping culture: The role of Bulgarian sports governing bodies. *Sport in Society*, 9(2), 252–268.

Glynn, M.A., & Abzug, R. (2002). Institutionalizing identity: Symbolic isomorphism and organizational names. *Academy of Management Journal*, 45(1), 267–280.

Gowthorp, L., Greenhow, A., & O'Brien, D. (2016). An interdisciplinary approach in identifying the legitimate regulator of anti-doping in sport: The case of the Australian Football League. *Sport Management Review*, 19(1), 48–60.

Greenwood, R., Oliver, C., Suddaby, R., & Sahlin-Andersson, K. (2008). *The Sage handbook of organizational institutionalism*. Thousand Oaks, CA: Sage.

Greenwood, R., Raynard, M., Kodeih, F., Micelotta, E.R., & Lounsbury, M. (2011). Institutional complexity and organizational responses. *The Academy of Management Annals*, 5(1), 317–371.

Haack, P., Schilke, O., & Zucker, L. (2020). Legitimacy revisited: Disentangling propriety, validity, and consensus. *Journal of Management Studies*. https://doi.org/10.1111/joms.12615

Hamilton, E.A. (2006). An exploration of the relationship between loss of legitimacy and the sudden death of organizations. *Group & Organization Management*, 31(3), 327–358.

Hanstad, D.V. (2008). Drug scandal and organizational change within the International Ski Federation: A figurational approach. *European sport management quarterly*, 8(4), 379–398.

Hanstad, D.V., & Houlihan, B. (2015). Strengthening global anti-doping policy through bilateral collaboration: The example of Norway and China. *International Journal of Sport Policy and Politics*, 7(4), 587–604.

Heinze, K.L., & Lu, D. (2017). Shifting responses to institutional change: The National Football League and player concussions. *Journal of Sport Management*, 31(5), 497–513.

Henning, A.D., & Dimeo, P. (2015). Questions of fairness and anti-doping in US cycling: The contrasting experiences of professionals and amateurs. *Drugs: Education, Prevention and Policy*, 22(5), 400–409.

Henning, A.D., & Dimeo, P. (2019). Perceptions of legitimacy, attitudes and buy-in among athlete groups: A cross-national qualitative investigation providing practical solutions. The World Anti-Doping Agency. Retrieved from https://www.wadaama.org/en/resources/social-science/

Heugens, P.P., & Lander, M.W. (2009). Structure! Agency! (and other quarrels): A metaanalysis of institutional theories of organization. *Academy of Management Journal*, 52(1), 61–85.

Holm, P. (1995). The dynamics of institutionalization: Transformation processes in Norwegian fisheries. *Administrative Science Quarterly*, 40(3), 398–422.

Houlihan, B. (2009). Mechanisms of international influence on domestic elite sport policy. *International Journal of Sport Policy*, 1(1), 51–69.

Jepperson, R. (1991). Institutions, institutional effects, and institutionalism: The new institutionalism in organizational analysis (pp. 143–163). Chicago, IL: University of Chicago press.

Kostova, T., & Zaheer, S. (1999). Organizational legitimacy under conditions of complexity: The case of the multinational enterprise. *Academy of Management Review*, 24(1), 64–81.

Kraatz, M.S., & Block, E.S. (2008). Organizational implications of institutional pluralism. In R. Greenwood, C. Oliver, T. Lawrence & R. Meyer (Eds.), *The Sage handbook of organizational institutionalism* (pp. 243–275). Thousand Oaks, CA: Sage.

Linsley, P., & Kajuter, P. (2008). Restoring reputation and repairing legitimacy: A case study of impression management in response to a major risk event at Allied Irish Banks plc. *International Journal of Financial Services Management*, 3(1), 65–82.

Lock, D., Filo, K., Kunkel, T., & Skinner, J.L. (2015). The development of a framework to capture perceptions of sport organizations legitimacy. *Journal of Sport Management*, 29(4), 362–379.

MacLean, T.L., & Behnam, M. (2010). The dangers of decoupling: The relationship between compliance programs, legitimacy perceptions, and institutionalized misconduct. *Academy of Management Journal*, 53(6), 1499–1520.

McDermott, V. (2015). The war on drugs in sport: Moral panics and organizational legitimacy. London, UK: Routledge.

McDermott, V., Henne, K., & Connor, J. (2013). *Legitimating the fight? Questions about cross-cultural perspectives on anti-doping strategies in the Pacific, TASA 2013: Reflections, intersections and aspirations* (pp. 1–12). Caulfield, Australia: The Australian Sociological Association (TASA).

Merriam, S.B. (1998). *Qualitative research and case study applications in education, revised and expanded from 'Case study research in education'.* San Francisco, CA: Jossey-Bass.

Meyer, J.W., & Rowan, B. (1977). Institutionalized organizations: Formal structure as myth and ceremony. *American Journal of Sociology*, 83(2), 340–363.

Ortiz, D., Myers, D., Walls, E., & Diaz, M.E. (2005). Where do we stand with newspaper data? *Mobilization: An International Quarterly*, 10(3), 397–419.

Oliver, C. (1991). Strategic responses to institutional complexity. *Academy of Management Review*, 16, 145–179. 10.5465/amr.1991.4279002.

Overbye, M., & Wagner, U. (2014). Experiences, attitudes and trust: An inquiry into elite athletes' perception of the whereabouts reporting system. *International Journal of Sport Policy and Politics*, 6(3), 407–428.

Pache, A.C., & Santos, F. (2010). When worlds collide: The internal dynamics of organizational responses to conflicting institutional demands. *Academy of Management Review*, 35(3), 455–476.

Pache, A.C., & Santos, F. (2013). Inside the hybrid organization: Selective coupling as a response to competing institutional logics. *Academy of Management Journal*, 56(4), 972–1001.

Powell, W.W., & Colyvas, J.A. (2008). Microfoundations of institutional theory. In S. Clegg, C. Hardy, T. Lawrence, & W. Nord (Eds.), *The Sage handbook of organization studies* (pp. 276–298). London, UK: Sage.

Qvarfordt, A., Hoff, D., Bäckström, Å., & Ahmadi, N. (2019). From fighting the bad to protecting the good: Legitimation strategies in WADA's athlete guides. *Performance Enhancement & Health, 7*(1–2), 100–147.

Raynard, M. (2016). Deconstructing complexity: Configurations of institutional complexity and structural hybridity. *Strategic Organization, 14*(4), 310–335.

Read, D., Skinner, J., Lock, D., & Houlihan, B. (2019). Legitimacy driven change at the world anti-doping agency. *International Journal of Sport Policy and Politics, 11*(2), 233–245.

Ritchie, I., & Jackson, G. (2014). Politics and 'shock': Reactionary anti-doping policy objectives in Canadian and international sport. *International Journal of Sport Policy and Politics, 6*(2), 195–212.

Scott, W.R. (2008). *Institutions and organizations: Ideas and interests*. London, UK: Sage.

Seo, M.G., & Creed, W.D. (2002). Institutional contradictions, praxis, and institutional change: A dialectical perspective. *Academy of Management Review, 27*(2), 222–247.

Silverman, D. (2015). *Interpreting qualitative data*. London, UK: Sage.

Skille, E.Å., Hanstad, D.V., & Tjernsbekk, P.A. (2011). The institutionalization of National Anti-doping Work after the introduction of the World Anti-Doping Code. *International Journal of Applied Sports Sciences, 23*(2).

Starke, C., & Flemming, F. (2017). Who is responsible for doping in sports? The attribution of responsibility in the German print media. *Communication & Sport, 5*(2), 245–262.

Staw, B.M., & Epstein, L.D. (2000). What bandwagons bring: Effects of popular management techniques on corporate performance, reputation, and CEO pay. *Administrative Science Quarterly, 45*(3), 523–556.

Suchman, M.C. (1995). Managing legitimacy: Strategic and institutional approaches. *Academy of Management Review, 20*(3), 571–610.

Suddaby, R., Bitektine, A., & Haack, P. (2017). Legitimacy. *Academy of Management Annals, 11*(1), 451–478.

Thornton, P.H., & Ocasio, W. (1999). Institutional logics and the historical contingency of power in organizations: Executive succession in the higher education publishing industry, 1958–1990. *American Journal of Sociology, 105*(3), 801–843.

Toohey, K., & Beaton, A. (2017). International cross-sector social partnerships between sport and governments: The World Anti-Doping Agency. *Sport Management Review, 20*(5), 483–496.

Tost, L.P. (2011). An integrative model of legitimacy judgments. *Academy of Management Review, 36*(4), 686–710.

Wagner, U. (2010). The international cycling union under siege—anti-doping and the biological passport as a mission impossible? *European Sport Management Quarterly, 10*(3), 321–342.

Wagner, U. (2011). Towards the construction of the world anti-doping agency: Analyzing the approaches of FIFA and the IAAF to doping in sport. *European Sport Management Quarterly, 11*(5), 445–470.

Walsh, J., & McAllister-Spooner, S.M. (2011). Analysis of the image repair discourse in the Michael Phelps controversy. *Public Relations Review, 37*(2), 157–162.

Weber, M. (1978). *Economy and society: An outline of interpretive sociology* (p. 1). Berkeley: University of California Press.

Westphal, J.D., & Zajac, E.J. (2001). Decoupling policy from practice: The case of stock repurchase programs. *Administrative Science Quarterly, 46*(2), 202–228.

Woolway, T., Lazuras, L., Barkoukis, V., & Petróczi, A. (2020). 'Doing what is right and doing it right': A mapping review of athletes' perception of anti-doping legitimacy. *International Journal of Drug Policy, 84*.

Wu, Z., & Salomon, R. (2016). Does imitation reduce the liability of foreignness? Linking distance, isomorphism, and performance. *Strategic Management Journal, 37*(12), 2441–2462.

Zimmerman, M.A., & Zeitz, G.J. (2002). Beyond survival: Achieving new venture growth by building legitimacy. *Academy of Management Review, 27*(3), 414–431.

Zucker, L.G. (1977). The role of institutionalization in cultural persistence. *American Sociological Review, 42*(5), 726–743.

Chapter 3

The creation of the World Anti-Doping Agency

Before progressing to discuss more recent events in anti-doping, it is necessary to firstly inspect the conditions that led to WADA's creation to fully understand its legitimacy and effectiveness. By analysing the legitimacy debate that followed the 1998 Festina scandal about the appropriateness of the IOC to regulate drugs in sport, it is possible to see which actors were able to successfully influence the institutional change that led to WADA's creation, and which actors were suppressed. It is also possible to explore whether stakeholders reached a consensus about the validity of WADA as a new institution. This chapter will go on to establish that within the field of Olympic sport, there was a lack of consensus about the legitimacy of an independent anti-doping organisation in sport, particularly from IOC executives who wished to maintain control of anti-doping regulation. However, due to the Salt Lake City Olympic bidding scandal preceding the Lausanne Conference, the IOC's perceived ethical integrity was at an all-time low. The perceived lack of integrity bled into other issues, including anti-doping, which meant that the IOC lacked legitimacy to stop governments inserting themselves into anti-doping regulation. Consequently, WADA was a proverbial house built on sand as the organisation emerged from a compromise. The organisation's legitimacy and lack of behavioural support since has partly stemmed from the lack of consensus that characterised its creation.

Olympic sport in the 1990s was characterised by a long series of continued drugs scandals, culminating in 1998 with the so-called Festina scandal. These scandals undermined the legitimacy of the IOC to regulate anti-doping. In response, the IOC organised the Lausanne Conference in February 1999 to reassert its control over anti-doping under the guise of the proposed Olympic Movement Anti-Doping Agency (OMADA), a non-independent global anti-doping agency headed by IOC officials. As this chapter will go on to discuss, the outcome of the Lausanne Conference was arguably the most important institutional juncture in the history of anti-doping. At the Lausanne Conference, it was agreed in principle that responsibility for regulating anti-doping in IOC-recognised sports would be transferred to a new independent organisation and not OMADA. The decision to create an independent organisation set in motion processes that would lead to the development and establishment of WADA in 1999. The creation of WADA meant that, regardless of individual judgements about the importance of anti-doping, there were now strong suppressor factors applied to organisations and individuals involved with Olympic sports to support (at least publicly) the activities of the new organisation. Therefore, understanding which judgements were successfully promoted during the legitimacy debate around WADA's creation provides insight into the initial validation of WADA as a basis for discussion of the following cases in chapters four to nine.

Accordingly, we begin the chapter by providing an overview of the state of anti-doping prior to the creation of WADA, the events preceding the Festina scandal and details of the Lausanne Conference. The second section details the key periods of instability and legitimacy debates regarding the IOC's regulation of anti-doping between the Festina affair in 1998 and WADA's launch in 1999 debate. The first identified period follows the comments of former IOC President Juan Antonio Samaranch (1980–2001) in July 1998, to reduce restrictions on doping. The second period is the Lausanne Conference in February 1999, and the final period of debate starts in Summer 1999 when the IOC first proposed an anti-doping code through to the Sydney Summit in November 1999. The final section presents the findings of the analysis under four key points. Firstly, government intervention covers how activist governments presented a collective opposition to the IOC challenging its performance. Secondly, in commercial power, the ability of wealthy International Federations (IFs) to reject mandatory two-year suspensions is discussed. Thirdly, the IOC's failed resistance is introduced as the Executive Committee tried to resist legitimacy challenges but was ineffective in utilising these. Fourthly, the ability of the IOC to reach an effective compromise on anti-doping regulation and the implications for WADA are considered. These discussion points contribute to the key message in this chapter, that WADA's legitimacy as an institution and source of institutional pressures was weakly validated. The weak validation reflects a lack of consensus about the value of WADA and can help us understand the challenges the organisation has since faced in trying to gain behavioural support from signatories.

A decade of doping scandals

Prior to the creation of WADA, anti-doping regulation in Olympic sports was characterised by a lack of effort on behalf of officials and a lack of clarity as each IF had its own anti-doping policies and requirements (Houlihan, 2002). Developments in pharmaceutical enhancement of performance achieved during World War II contributed to an increasing problem with performance-enhancing drugs (PED) use in sport from the 1950s onwards. The problem of PED use was treated as a threat to the amateur ideals of Olympism where athletes should participate not to win, but for the wider benefits of sport (Gleaves, 2011; Gleaves & Llewellyn, 2014). Drug use in sport was regarded as a public image problem for the IOC, and apathy towards the issue led to fragmented and inadequate testing (Hunt, 2011). However, myriad factors including cold war politics, pharmaceutical advancements, the professionalisation of sport, improved sports medicine and commercialisation meant that through the 1960s, 1970s and 1980s drug use in sport became a more prominent and uncomfortable problem for the IOC that had previously relied on largely superficial measures (Houlihan, 2002).

Throughout the late 1980s and 1990s a series of events brought increasing attention to doping in sport. In 1988, Olympic 100-m champion Ben Johnson was disqualified and stripped off his victory after he tested positive for Stanozolol. Johnson's disqualification was a 'focussing event' (Ritchie & Jackson, 2014, p. 198) for the IOC and anti-doping policy and marked the start of a decade of doping scandals in the 1990s. Clear evidence began to emerge of state-sponsored doping in the German Democratic Republic after the fall of the Berlin Wall (Franke & Berendonk, 1997) as well as increasing evidence of widespread doping among Chinese athletes (Hunt, 2011). These high-profile scandals brought the IOC's reputation in regard to anti-doping management under further scrutiny (Waddington, 2016). In the same period, a handful of national governments from leading Olympic countries, such as the United Kingdom, Canada and Norway, began developing their own anti-doping activities in the early 1980s. By 1998 a small international network of governments from Europe, the Antipodes and North America concerned about doping in sport had begun to develop through international agreements and the Council of Europe (Houlihan, 2002; Waddington, 2016).

The year 1998 was a particularly bad year for doping stories as three-time swimming gold medallist at the 1996 Olympic Games Michelle Smith failed a doping test, baseball legend Mark McGwire admitted to the use of (then legal) steroid precursors and Australian customs officials made a major seizure of human growth hormones from Chinese swimmers entering the country. The tipping point was the Festina scandal at the 1998 Tour de France where French border officials arrested Team Festina soigneur, Willy Voet, for possession of a wide range of PEDs and associated paraphernalia. Voet's arrest led to further arrests at the Tour involving riders, doctors and managers. The Festina scandal was significant because of the already growing intervention of government border agencies into the previously autonomous issue of drugs in sport. The continued corruption of Olympic sports and increasing government involvement in anti-doping efforts leading up to the Festina scandal meant that it acted as a final straw for a growing sense of disillusionment by certain national officials (Dimeo & Møller, 2018). Wagner and Pedersen (2014) argued that the Festina scandal was especially critical because, following Ben Johnson, the IOC had created a discourse of winning the war on drugs. The Festina scandal demonstrated the opposite.

In response to growing criticisms of the IOC's attitude to anti-doping, IOC president Juan Antonio Samaranch declared that the Lausanne Conference would be held in February 1999 to provide 'a clear definition of doping' ('Samaranch calls for world conference', 1998, July 27). It has been argued that the IOC's decision to hold the Lausanne Conference was motivated by a need to be seen to be doing something rather than proactively trying to improve anti-doping policy (Ritchie & Jackson, 2014). Before the Lausanne Conference, in December 1998 it was discovered that members of the IOC had been involved in a vote-buying scandal for the upcoming Salt Lake City Olympics in 2002. IOC members were revealed to have taken bribes in exchanges for voting for Salt Lake City to host the 2002 Winter Olympics. In January 1999, six IOC members were recommended for expulsion due to corruption. The vote-buying scandal was particularly damaging to the IOC because it directly contradicted the ethical principles around which the Olympics crafted and marketed its identity (Glynn, Watkiss, Raffaelli, & Blyler, 2012).

   The combination of the bidding and Festina scandals represented a significant threat to the legitimacy of the IOC (Hunt, 2011). Consequently, the Lausanne Conference was hijacked by a select group of government officials who used it as an opportunity to challenge the IOC by demanding the creation of a new independent anti-doping agency (Ferstle, 2001). Government officials argued that the IOC was morally bankrupt (Smith, 1999a, February 5) and could not be trusted with policing doping in sport. Despite the IOC's attempt to construct the conference in a manner that minimised opportunity for dissent, the conference led to a number of unplanned outcomes stipulated in the Lausanne Declaration (Waddington, 2016). Most prominently, the revised Lausanne Declaration on Doping in Sport (1999) declared that an 'Independent International Anti-Doping Agency' (p. 2) would be created. Subsequently, WADA was created as a hybrid organisation between sport and government officials, with the purpose of creating a universal anti-doping policy for IOC-recognised sports and regulating implementation of the policy. As Hanstad, Smith, and Waddington (2008) concluded, rather than taking back control, the IOC helped 'institutionalize the role of governments at the very heart of anti-doping policy' (p. 241).

   Casini (2009) referred to state involvement as the 'partial nationalisation' (p. 439) of anti-doping and cited the harmonisation of anti-doping efforts and the introduction of 'administrative law-type principles' (p. 444) as positive outcomes of WADA. However, there is disagreement about whether WADA is free from IOC interference. Dimeo and Møller (2018) noted that the IOC was able to install an IOC member as the inaugural head of WADA, undermining the agency's perceived independence. The IOC also ensured 50% of Executive Committee positions were for Olympic movement officials. More critically, Hunt, Dimeo, and Jedlicka (2012) concluded that the conference missed the opportunity to review the rationale for anti-doping meaning WADA was 'defensive, traditionalist and out-of-touch with reality' (p. 58) reinforcing the IOC's original approach to regulation.

Considering the well-established conclusion that the Lausanne Conference led to institutional change within the field of anti-doping (e.g., Hanstad et al., 2008), there is utility to discussing the events surrounding the creation of WADA from a multi-level legitimacy perspective. This analysis can elucidate which stakeholders were dominated and suppressed in this period to understand the motivations behind the legitimacy challenges WADA has faced since. Therefore, it is an appropriate case to study the legitimacy of WADA. The following section will now present the key periods of legitimacy debate identified in the analysis.

Key periods of instability

Inspection of newspaper coverage helped identify three key periods of instability pertaining to the creation of WADA occurring between the Festina scandal and WADA's inaugural meeting. In these periods there is inspection and debate of the IOC's legitimacy as chief regulator of anti-doping as field members launched verbal and behavioural challenges. These periods therefore provide an insight into the level of consensus between members of the anti-doping field at the time.

The first key period followed the Festina scandal, and more specifically the comments of IOC President Juan Antonio Samaranch in late July 1998. The Union Cycliste Internationale (International Cycling Union; UCI) came under great scrutiny as professional cycling teams: Team Festina and TVM were both implicated in socially organised doping at the 1998 Tour de France. The situation was further complicated as doctors and former riders came forward about the endemic use of PEDs in professional cycling. The UCI struggled as Tour sponsors questioned whether to maintain their financial obligations (Evagora, 1998, July 21) and Tour riders attempted to stage a boycott due to the involvement of French police in anti-doping. At the time newspaper coverage focused on the UCI and the cycling 'omerta' (the culture of silence about drug use in professional cycling). It was the comments of IOC President Samaranch in Spanish newspaper El Mundo at the end of July that drew the IOC into the debate. Samaranch proclaimed: 'Doping (now) is everything that, firstly, is harmful to an athlete's health and, secondly, artificially augments his performance. If it's just the second case, for me that's not doping. If it's the first case, it is' (McMillan, 1998, July 28). Samaranch's comments drew legitimacy challenges in relation to the IOC's commitment to anti-doping from sport ministers and athletes. Part of the IOC's subsequent attempt to rectify this was by announcing the Lausanne Conference. The IOC may have still held the Lausanne Conference following the Festina scandal, but had Samaranch not said 'the most extraordinary thing anyone has ever said in elite sport' as Australia's Federal Sports Minister Andrew Thomson claimed ('Thomson appalled', 1998, July 28), the IOC may have been judged as more concerned with anti-doping.

The second period that encouraged legitimacy debate and challenges was the Lausanne Conference in early February 1999. The conference provided an opportunity for usually separate national governments' representatives to unite and project legitimacy challenges at the IOC. These were constituted of both pragmatic (e.g., the IOC's poor record on doping regulation) and moral (e.g., the ethical integrity of the IOC Executive Committee) concerns. Governments' representatives also drew upon Samaranch's comments following the Festina scandal as well as the 2002 Salt Lake City Winter Olympic bidding scandal which was fresh in the mind of conference attendees. Taken together, these scandals painted an image of an incompetent and morally bankrupt organisation. However, the conference also gave the IOC an instant opportunity to respond to the criticisms. At the end of the conference, the IOC continued to experience disapproval due to its decision to retreat on compulsory two-year bans for all anti-doping violations in Olympic sports. The *exceptional circumstances rule*, as it was termed, was viewed as a concession to the affluent football and cycling governing bodies. The rule allowed organisations to reduce bans for anti-doping rule violations (ADRVs) in what the IFs determined were exceptional circumstances, essentially creating a legal loophole.

The third period in the latter half of 1999 followed the proposed draft of how the new independent organisation would be structured, the first anti-doping code the IOC attempted to promote and the Sydney Summit in late 1999. At the end of the Lausanne Conference, the Lausanne Declaration was signed. Although the IOC agreed to an independent anti-doping agency, the conference failed to determine how this should be structured or governed, and the IOC was set the task of designing an organisation that was acceptable to all sources. The IOC's initial proposals were viewed as legally and practically inadequate (Salvado, 1999, August 5). The final proposal put forward was better received, and Australian authorities organised the Sydney Summit on 14 November 1999 to connect government ministers from around the world to debate the IOC proposals. Given Australia's involvement in catching Chinese athletes with PEDs in 1998 and its attempt to make the 2000 Sydney Olympic Games in Australia the 'cleanest games ever', the Australian public were disappointed that the Minister for Sport, Amanda Vanstone, had not attended the Lausanne Conference. Instead, the head of the Australian Anti-Doping Agency attended the conference. In what appeared to be an attempt to regain credit, the Sydney Summit was arranged. Coverage of the Summit was dominated by the feud between American general John McCaffrey, who believed the IOC's proposals were inadequate due to the inclusion of Olympic officials in the governing body, and Australian IOC member John Coates, who believed America did not have the authority to challenge the IOC on anti-doping matters because of the country's historically lax approach to anti-doping. Consequently, McCaffrey launched challenges at the IOC, but ultimately the governments present at the summit gave their support to WADA.

Based on patterns across the three periods, four main discussion points emerged: (1) government intervention, (2) commercial power, (3) failed resistance and (4) effective compromise that are now presented.

Government intervention

Government intervention captures the unexpected (by the IOC) legitimacy challenges launched by ministers from the European Union (EU), United States, Australia and Canada following the Festina scandal. The Festina scandal and Samaranch's comments appear to have signalled to government ministers that the IOC was failing to regulate anti-doping in Olympic sports. Each government had specific reasons for valuing anti-doping in sport, or at least ensuring that the image of sport remained clean. The EU nations were unified by a perception that the European roots of the Olympics meant they should protect the integrity of the games and that sport had a unique societal influence across European nations (Council of Europe, 1998, November 5). The United States saw doping in sport as an extension of the domestic war on drugs (Executive Office of the White House, 1998, November 17). Australia was due to host the 2000 Olympic Summer Games in Sydney and was heavily invested in ensuring it was perceived as clean. Finally, Canada was trying to position itself as a world leader in anti-doping following its response to Ben Johnson's doping (Canadian Olympic Association, 1998, December 16).

These governments challenged the legitimacy of the IOC on pragmatic and moral grounds. It is clear following the Festina scandal that these governments perceived Samaranch's comments on doping as detrimental to their efforts. For example, Australian Federal Sports Minister Andrew Thomson expressed frustration: 'It's appalling that we are here doing our best to fight against drugs and our politicians should be undermined by people beyond our borders' ("Thomson appalled over Samaranch remarks", 1998, July 28). Similarly, Diane Jones-Konihowski, committee member of the Canadian Centre for Ethics in Sport responsible for anti-doping in Canada, argued: 'I guess when I read it, you really question at my level why we're working so hard, and the control lies at that high level. It's really disheartening' ('U.S. track stars', 1998, July 28). Jim Ferguson, head of the Australian Sports Commission, more bluntly pointed out: 'If we're only worried about drugs if they hurt health then you open up flood of cheating' (Moore, 1998, July 29). These comments articulated that Samaranch's remarks were harmful to the actives and self-interest of governmental organisations and anti-doping bodies.

Government representatives also challenged the IOC on moral grounds, due to the behaviour of IOC President Samaranch. For example, former British Olympic Association head Sir Arthur Gold claimed: 'These are very unwise remarks by the IOC President and I disagree totally with them. To use drugs is to cheat whether they damage your health or not' ('Samaranch calls for world conference', 1998, July 27). The response to Samaranch's comments demonstrated the impact individuals within an organisation can have upon the legitimacy of an entire organisation.

Moral challenges expressed by government representatives suggested that the IOC was failing to protect the 'values' of sport following the Salt Lake City scandal. Moral challenges transcended the issue of anti-doping and directly targeted the IOC. There are numerous examples of how the Festina scandal and ensuing events led ministers to question the IOC. Prior to the Lausanne Conference, General McCaffrey remarked:

> I've watched with enormous dismay the loss of legitimacy of the IOC over this issue. I really believe it's outrageous that collectively they failed to recognize they have a trust, not a tenure. The global community must have that corrected. And I'm not sure that they are capable of correcting it themselves.
> (Fish, 1999, January 26)

His comments suggest that both the Salt Lake City and the Festina scandals diminished the IOC's legitimacy in respect to more than just its ability to regulate anti-doping. Once the conference began, this line of challenge continued. Tony Banks on behalf of the EU representatives commented on the IOC's governance following the Salt Lake City scandal:

> We do expect the IOC to reform its structure. It's not the sort of structure that should enter the 21st century. Juan Antonio Samaranch understands that. We believe in the principles of the Olympic movement, but at the moment it is looking rather sad, and rather soured, and rather sullied.
> (Rowbottom, 1999, February 3)

Others ministers linked the doping problem to the higher values of sport, Irish Minister John Treacy said, 'The integrity of sport is at stake'; and Danish Minister Elsebeth Gerner Nielsen stated, 'It is the hour of destiny for the Olympic movement' (Dobbin, 1999, February 2) and suggested, 'The IOC should consider the possibility of preparing ethical accounts as a supplement to the impressive financial accounts' (Fish, 1999, February 3).

At the Conference, government representatives repeatedly criticised the proposed OMADA because it was judged to be too dependent on the IOC and, therefore, conflicted in its capacity to regulate anti-doping. For example, the Belgium Minister spoke for the EU nations: 'The European ministers stress they have the strongest reserve over the composition of the international anti-doping agency as presented in documents we have seen' (McCullough, 1999, February 2). British Minister Tony Banks added:

> It is our unanimous opinion that we cannot at present accept the composition of the agency. We ask that the principle of the agency being set up is accepted but that its composition and functions be subject of urgent consultation with the European Union and other interested bodies.
> (McCullough, 1999, February 4)

Numerous government ministers lined up to reiterate the need for independence – if the new organisation was to perform successfully. Francisco Villar, Spanish Secretary of State for Sports argued: 'The agency must not depend on the IOC. It must be independent' (Fish, 1999, February 3). Likewise, Danish Minister Nielsen echoed: 'The proposal of an international agency to govern and test internationally against doping deserves further consideration. But such an agency must, however, be completely independent and transparent' (McCullough, 1999, February 2). Italian Sports minister Giovanna Melandri specified: 'The agency should be truly independent from the IOC' (Casert, 1999, February 2) whilst General Barry McCaffrey, director of the US Drug Policy Office offered: 'The Olympic anti-drug and doping programme should be overseen by a separately established drugs testing and oversight agency' ('European Community', 1999, February 2). This reflected Otto Schily, the German interior minister and EU head's call that 'the European Union should speak with one voice in the fight against doping to lend more force to its demands at international conferences' ('EU ministers call', 1999, January 18).

Questions at the conference continued towards the impact of the exceptional circumstances rule that the IOC introduced in the Lausanne Declaration to satisfy certain IFs. As Tony Banks highlighted, 'The way that it's done at the moment has provided an enormous loophole. It is both minimalist and permissive. It undermines the proposal. Some people here believe the declaration has weakened rather than strengthened anti-doping initiatives' (Mackay, 1999, February 5). Australian Federal Sports Minister Jackie Kelly reflected on the proposal: 'We have concerns about the operation of the exceptional circumstances clauses. A clear definition is required for consistent application otherwise the impact of the two-year minimum sanction could be severely watered down' ('Sydney summit', 1999, February 6). Additionally, Finnish Minister Suvi-Anne Siimes reasoned: 'The sanctions must be substantial and unequivocal. The athlete's right to practise his or her profession cannot be a reason to vitiate the penalty imposed. The rules of the game are clear elsewhere' (McCullough, 1999, February 2). These comments reflect a general judgement from government representatives that the exceptional circumstances rule was detrimental to the work of anti-doping within their countries and was consequently illegitimate.

Even after the conference, government ministers continued to express criticisms reflective of their negative judgements of the IOC's legitimacy. Otto Schily suggested an 'Olympic boycott by European Union countries if the IOC fails to go forward on reform' (Hersh, 1999, March 15) and French Sports Minister Marie-George Buffet said that the outcomes of the Lausanne Conference were 'non-negotiable' ('EU ministers insist', 1999, March 15). When the IOC did initially propose a draft anti-doping code and structure for WADA, it faced further challenges for not reflecting the Lausanne Declaration, particularly from Australian commentators concerned about the approaching Sydney Olympics. Australian Olympic Committee legal adviser Simon Rofe asserted:

> If the IOC continues to adopt its previous anachronistic and high-handed approach without the recognition of submissions at the anti-doping conference, and particularly from the international federations, then we will not have a code worth looking at or even trying to implement. I've got no idea why the IOC is acting like this and that's the disappointing part.
>
> (Salvado, 1999, August 5)

Rofe's position was echoed by Australian IOC member John Coates who said:

> I have told President Samaranch that the drafting of the code fails to properly address critical terms and elements such as a proper definition of 'doping' and trafficking. Further, the code does not adequately address out-of-competition testing and does not contain any provision permitting therapeutic use by athletes of otherwise prohibited substances. Importantly, the sampling and testing procedures described in the code do not accord with world's best practice.
>
> ('Australian Olympic chief', 1999, September 8)

McCaffrey also challenged the proposed structure of WADA on the grounds that it did not reflect the Lausanne Declaration: 'It doesn't meet the criteria a bunch of us put on the table. As we read the IOC proposal, it falls short of the mark. The agency is not independent, and there is not sufficient accountability' (Shipley, 1999, September 16). A statement from the EU corroborated this point declaring: 'The agency should be genuinely transparent and independent' (Ames, 1999, October 19).

By the time of the Sydney Summit, however, the IOC faced fewer challenges, due in part to an agreement between the EU and the IOC. The new head of the EU Sports Commission, Viviane Reding, had originally stated: 'We want an agency that does not depend on the IOC' (Ames, 1999, October 19). However, she later retracted this point after a meeting with Samaranch which determined that the EU would have two representatives on the board, expressing: 'The EU wants to participate for a very simple reason. The sports world is an important part of the social component of Europe, most of all for the young people' ('EU to participate', 1999, November 2). In contrast, McCaffrey continued to voice his negative judgements of the proposals, for example: 'How can it be called independent when its chairman [Pound] has already been appointed before a board meeting' ('Olympic delegate rebuffs', 1999, November 15). At the summit, he added, 'It looks to us as though it will be dominated by the IOC. That, to us, is unacceptable' (Corder, 1999a, November 15). It appears that the government representatives that presented a consensus at the Lausanne Conference that forced concessions from the IOC were no longer united at the Sydney Summit, and the United States alone was unable to effectively challenge the legitimacy of the IOC.

In summary, there was an apparent consensus in legitimacy judgements between the small but powerful national governments in the field of anti-doping. The judgements expressed by government officials highlighted that the IOC was lacking both perceived pragmatic and moral legitimacy which then impacted perceptions of the proposed OMADA. The lack of perceived legitimacy across two dimensions may have been critical as national government representatives did not perceive a social or personal benefit from the IOC regulating anti-doping efforts and therefore rejected the IOC-supported OMADA.

Commercial power

Commercial power captures how media sports (Maennig, 2014), such as football, cycling and tennis, characterised by financial stability and wealth from sponsorship and television rights were able to reject proposals for mandatory two-year suspensions for all ADRVs. Media sport representatives argued that a two-year suspension could not be upheld in court, because such sanctions were far more severe in some sporting careers than others. Team athletes would not be able to train in this period compared to individual athletes, and a two-year ban in some sports (e.g., football) was a far larger period of an athlete's career than in other sports (e.g., shooting). This judgement reflected elements of pragmatic and moral consideration as it was perceived as the wrong thing to do for sport.

Prior to the Lausanne Conference, the IOC convened a meeting with the 35 IFs of the Summer and Winter Olympic Games at the end of November 1998 in an attempt to gain their support. The IOC proposed OMADA as a solution to the problem of variation between anti-doping regulations across sports. As IOC Medical Commission Chairman Prince Alexandre de Merode suggested, 'This agency [OMADA] will make us stronger than before. To be united is a key success of the anti-doping fight. We all have to be unified in this battle' (Wilson, 1998, August 20). Following the attempts of President Samaranch to unify all IFs behind his proposed OMADA before the Lausanne Conference, there was clear evidence of the International Federation of Association Football (FIFA) and the UCI's willingness to challenge the IOC. For example, FIFA Medical Committee chairman Michel D'Hooghe stated in objection to mandatory two-year suspensions that 'I can only tell you that FIFA will never change its opinion on this. Even if FIFA stands alone, it is old and big enough to take care of itself' (Christie 1999, January 5). Media sports representatives justified their objections based on arguments related to employment regulations. For example, D'Hooghe argued, 'It's far too easy to say something and have the first lawyer move in and call it illegal when somebody is robbed of his job for two years' (Christie, 1999, January 5). UCI President Hein Verbruggen presented a similar argument:

A uniform suspension brings discrimination of one sport against the other because a suspension of one year or even less will hit one athlete more severely than a suspension of four years in another sport. An athlete, for financial reasons and on principle, will never accept a suspension which is in fact a ban for life … they have nothing to lose and a lawsuit is the only possibility for them to come back.

(Magnay, 1999, January 29)

Evidently, prior to the Lausanne Conference, media sports had negatively judged the legitimacy of the IOC's proposals. Notably these evaluators do not cite their own sports when arguing against mandatory two-year bans which may be an attempt to appear more objective and disguise any pragmatic self-interest.

Challenges to the IOC's legitimacy continued prior to and throughout the Lausanne Conference along the same lines of previous argument. D'Hooghe re-iterated FIFA's unwillingness to compromise on its objections to mandatory suspensions, and when questioned about potential expulsion from the Olympics proclaimed: 'If that's the point of departure there will be no discussion possible. FIFA will never bow to that' (Casert, 1999, January 26). On the same issue of Olympic expulsion, FIFA President Sepp Blatter bluntly stated, 'If that happened, we will fight' ('Doping summit impossible', 1999, February 3). In regard to being dictated to about how to manage anti-doping, International Swimming Federation (FINA) Secretary Gunnar Werner said, 'It is not necessary that all federations use the same points. Some may use some points, some may use all' (Casert, 1999, February 1). Media sports representatives continued to question the legal defensibility of mandatory two-year suspensions as Verbruggen con-tended, 'As soon as you want to impose a minimum of two years, you are going to run from court to court' (Casert, 1999, February 3). Verbruggen also drew upon the lack of finance to defend these suspensions in court arguing, 'Longer sanctions will cause a rush from athletes to civil courts with risks for claims that we cannot afford. We don't have the finance' (Casert, 1999, February 3). D'Hooghe used a previous case from athletics where a four-year anti-doping suspension was reduced by a court for violating legal rights stating, 'They [the IOC] should have learned from this. So let us be realistic' (Casert, 1999, January 29).

In addition to legal arguments, there was the justification of the unfairness of two-year suspensions by highlighting the specific nature of team sports. For example, FIFA President Sepp Blatter explained: 'Distinction should be made and different circumstances should be taken into account' ('Doping summit impossible', 1999, February 3). Blatter later added, 'Professional and team sports need exceptions. If you have a positive test in a team sport, can you suspend the whole team? Be realistic' ('Doping summit impossible', 1999, February 3). These comments were presented in a way that it is for the good of all team sports that two-year mandatory suspensions be waived which again suggests an attempt to appear objective in their judgement of legitimacy. Blatter's address to the conference sums up the notion of objectivity and speaking on behalf of others:

What we cannot accept, what causes us difficulties as well as to other federations, is the idea of a fixed sanction, that is a two-year suspension.

Every judge has the right and possibility of changing his sanction. But why don't we give this possibility to the judge who has to take such decisions at the level of the national federation.

(Marshallsea, 1999, February 4)

By suggesting it causes 'other federations' difficulties, Blatter is portraying his judgement as representative, not just self-interested, and by drawing upon judges, he is suggesting that legal objectivity is required.

Congruent with challenges prior to Lausanne, there appeared to be an attempt to use language related to morality to appear more objective and less driven by self-interest. For example, Verbruggen pointed out, 'Only those rules which you can apply as universal rules for everyone in equal circumstances are morally justified' (Casert, 1999, January 29). His use of the term *morally justified* gave his challenge a sense of objectivity. D'Hooghe followed a similar argument: 'It would be fundamental inequality. Two years might be 20% of a soccer player's career while it will only be 5% of somebody else's career. This big drive for equality creates the worst inequality' (Casert, 1999, January 29). By drawing upon issues of inequality D'Hooghe's challenge becomes a matter of moral beliefs and justice based on the interests of athletes rather than self-interest. It is apparent then that representatives of these organisations used specific language in morally justifying their judgements to appear more engaged than a simple decision of self-interest.

However, the motives of these challenges may not have been determined by consideration for the effectiveness of anti-doping but rather the need to protect their sports from outside interference. The comments of D'Hooghe at the end of conference are telling in understanding the motives for FIFA: 'Now we can continue to go our own way and deal with the doping issue the way we feel it should be done' (Casert, 1999, February 4). This statement would suggest that FIFA's ultimate goal was to maintain control of its anti-doping regulations, rather than ensuring anti-doping had a legally defendable suspension in place.

This section has again demonstrated the variety of competing legitimacy judgements in the field of anti-doping as well as exemplifying how more powerful organisations are able to maintain defiant positions. As the next section explores, the IOC used access to the Olympic Games in an attempt to coerce behavioural support for OMADA. Yet these media sports were financially stable enough to negate this pressure. Similarly, potential financial or reputational damage did not appear to be a major concern to these organisations.

Failed resistance

Failed resistance encompasses how the IOC used a combination of responses to actively resist legitimacy challenges from media sports and government representatives but was unsuccessful. By resisting challenges, it suggests that the IOC was unwilling or unable to accede to the arguments and judgements presented by IFs and governments.

We argue that the original comments of Samaranch in El Mundo were an attempt to influence anti-doping beliefs. Samaranch declared: 'Doping (now) is everything that, firstly, is harmful to an athlete's health and, secondly, artificially augments his performance. If it's just the second case, for me that's not doping. If it's the first case, it is' (McMillan, 1998, July 28). By suggesting that the boundaries of what constituted doping be reduced, he was attempting to influence the norms surrounding anti-doping in the Olympic movement. But as previously stated in 'Government intervention', his comments were met with widespread criticism suggesting he was trying to veil a step-down in anti-doping policy. In the following days, IOC officials attempted to reject the challenges by suggesting Samaranch had been misunderstood. For example, IOC Director General Francois Carrard asserted: 'He [Samaranch] never meant to give up the fight against doping or to launch himself a change of policy. There is no change in policy' (Wilson, 1998, July 28). Samaranch later clarified his comments dismissing that he wanted to change the definition of doping:

> I never said performance-enhancing drugs must be withdrawn from the list. I would like to ask the medical commission to review the list like they are doing from time to time. Maybe we need to put the list up to date. As for performance-enhancing drugs, there is not a single one that is not harming the health of the athletes. We will not withdraw one single performance-enhancing drug which we have on the list.
>
> (Wilson, 1998, August 20)

However, shortly after Samaranch's original comments, the IOC declared it would be hosting the Lausanne Conference. IOC officials were quick to highlight how the government officials who had criticised Samaranch could be brought into Olympic anti-doping positions, as IOC Executive Board member Jacques Rogge explained:

> We realised at the moment of the Tour de France in our fight against doping the sports would need the support of the governments. Only the governments have warrants, only the governments can search, can interrogate, can arrest and penalise the people who do not belong to the sports federations.
>
> (Salvado, 1998, July 29)

Michael Knight, who was head of the Sydney Olympic Games organising committee, supported this position: 'You are dependent on the activities of the police, customs officials, and others, so yes we're very happy for them to play a role. That's not to say that we want them strip-searching athletes as they arrive in Sydney' (Salvado, 1998, July 30). What is common between these quotes is that they imply that governments should be involved but only to an extent determined by the IOC. The IOC's desire for minimal government involvement is pointedly characterised by IOC Executive Committee member Dick Pound: 'We don't want governments running sport. We prefer that governments provide support for our anti-doping programmes' (Myers, 1998, September 14). This behaviour is typical of attempts to manipulate institutional pressures by co-opting the source of challenges into organisational structures (Oliver, 1991). The purpose of co-opting is for an organisation to benefit from the legitimacy granted from working with the challenger while simultaneously reducing the threat the challenger poses.

As highlighted under 'Commercial power' not all sport organisations would consent to backing OMADA going into the Lausanne Conference. Behind the IOC's attempt to recruit support was a more coercive threat of potential Olympic expulsion should IFs not want to be part of the solution. For example, IOC Executive Committee member and current IOC President Thomas Bach explained:

> I don't think we will have to threaten [the federations], but if the organizations refuse to cooperate and the world conference isn't a success, they will feel pressure from the IOC. Federations, who refuse, could lose their part of Olympic TV money. Sports, or at least some disciplines, could disappear out of the Olympic program.
>
> ('IOC official', 1998, November 13)

An anonymous leading IOC official was more restrained in stating: 'There are no threats. But an obligation is obviously implied and if you are not meeting it you are not part of the Olympic movement' (Fotheringham, 1998, November 28). Evidently, the IOC was leveraging access to the lucrative Olympic Games to dominate institutional pressures and legitimate OMADA.

The IOC was subject to a wide range of legitimacy challenges from government sports ministers at the Lausanne Conference. The ministers were there because of the IOC's attempt to co-opt governments into the Olympic processes without allowing them any real power. The reality was governments were able to reject IOC proposals and challenge the IOC around issues of independence and leadership. In response, the IOC defied the legitimacy challenges raised. For example, when the independence of an organisation involving the IOC was questioned, IOC executive Dick Pound asserted:

> They're going to have to live with that, because we are going to be part of any solution to the doping problem. We've been in it from the start, where 99% of the progress in doping has been as a result of the IOC involvement. And, in fact, without our involvement in something like that, without our willingness to put in money, it's not going to exist.
>
> (Edwards, 1999, February 3)

IOC Vice-President Anita DeFrantz used a similar line of argument: 'Cynics will say it's not independent, but someone has to fund it' (Wilson, 1999, February 1).

Other IOC officials were less diplomatic when the potential IOC leadership of a new organisation was questioned, for example, French Olympic Committee President Henri Serandour declared in regard to government ministers: 'They should not take the others for being naive and small people. They should stop giving us lessons. They want to appear whiter than white' ('US criticized', 1999, February 3). Prince De Merode echoed the sentiment of Serandour:

> It would be a terrible mistake to exclude experienced IOC members from this. I take offence that politicians don't trust me to chair this agency. Why should I trust politicians? Ask people in the streets if there is a great confidence in politicians. I have some doubts.
>
> (Wilson, 1999, February 2)

Some IOC officials directly targeted officials from the United States, for example, Jacques Rogge who would go on to succeed Samaranch as IOC President attacked the United States' previous efforts:

> As far as I know, the United States still has no anti-doping law today. The United States is a country where in professional sports you see a lack of real anti-doping rules, where you see that one of the biggest heroes, McGwire, is admitting taking androstenedione, which is forbidden in all other sports around the world.
>
> (Wilson, 1999, February 2)

Similarly, de Merode asserted: 'I'm surprised at the United States, coming in so late, having denied the existence of doping; then to come later and say it is not enough. You have to do more. That's incredible' (Christie, 1999a, February 4). It appears then that the IOC perceived discrediting and dismissing the legitimacy challenges as an appropriate response to managing its legitimacy.

Even following the Lausanne Conference, the IOC continued to defy legitimacy challenges based on its suggestions of how an independent anti-doping organisation would operate. The IOC's initial drafts of an anti-doping code and organisation were challenged for rejecting the agreements drawn up in the Lausanne declaration. For example, when the proposed code and design of WADA was challenged by Australian and American officials, Dick Pound countered: 'It ignores a lot of good work that has been done leading to an international consensus for the agency. That's what we promised at the world conference and that's what we've delivered' (Wilson, 1999, September 23). Furthermore, Jacques Rogge attacked General McCaffrey of America who had questioned the independence of WADA: 'If General McCaffrey is not happy, he better consult with the other governments who have given their approval. He should not point the finger at the IOC' (Wilson, 1999, September 23).

In summary, the IOC consistently avoided and defied the legitimacy challenges posed by governments, and we argue this response was ineffective.

Samaranch's early attempts to influence anti-doping beliefs were unsuccessful. For example, the IOC was unable to control all IFs as media sports dissented, failed to co-opt government involvement into OMADA on their terms, and attempts to dismiss challenges were ineffective in discrediting government ministers who were able to successfully validate the belief that an independent anti-doping agency was needed.

Effective compromise

The final discussion point of this chapter is effective compromise which develops how the IOC reverted from resisting challenges to the more passive response of compromising to avoid total loss of control over anti-doping. Submitting to all challenges from government representatives would have meant the IOC receding all control over anti-doping which would have presented an exceptional threat to the commercial viability of the Olympics should it expose widespread doping in other Olympic sports as witnessed in cycling (Hanstad et al., 2008). Reaching an appropriate compromise appeared to be the only way the IOC could suitably handle the challenges presented. Evidently, government representatives expected the IOC to relinquish control of anti-doping, and the IOC wanted to maintain autonomy over anti-doping. Given that the IOC lacked the legitimacy to validate OMADA, it had the remaining option to present concessions made by both IOC and its challengers as a win for anti-doping, thus, enabling the organisation to regain legitimacy.

Evidence of the IOC's increased willingness can be seen leading up to the Lausanne Conference as its attempts to manipulate IFs had failed. Prince de Merode as head of the IOC Medical Commission was at the front of growing recognition for compromise. For example, following FIFA, ITF and UCI rejecting mandatory sanctions Prince de Merode suggested: 'We will have a sentence like "can be reduced in exceptional cases". At that point, FIFA can be satisfied and tennis and cycling would be able to accept such a text' (Stanaway, 1999, January 30). He also tried to find alternatives to the mandatory two-year suspension including bans from major competitions:

> If they can't take part in big events, they won't be paid as much as before, and everyone will understand that they are punished. But they do not completely lose their opportunity to work. I think these sanctions can be applied without being reversed by the courts.
>
> (Longman, 1999, January 29)

Prince de Merode's position is a clear step-down from the original proposal that all IFs would have mandatory two-year suspensions and failure to agree could lead to Olympic expulsion.

The IOC's willingness to compromise on the exceptional circumstances rule was clear from other IOC members at the Lausanne Conference. For example,

Jacques Rogge rationalised the decision to introduce exceptional circumstances: 'You have to be reasonable. This is not a debate in black and white. You cannot compare athletes. Some careers span eight years, some span 20 years. Sanctions have to be adapted to that' (Casert, 1999, February 2). The compromise was portrayed as a success for anti-doping as John Coates exemplified:

> There won't be uniform sanctions across the sports. But the starting point is a very big improvement on where we were, because now the starting point is a two-year minimum for all sports, unless an athlete can show, on the balance of probabilities, that he or she fits within the specific exceptional category that has been approved for that sport.
>
> (Marshallsea, 1999, February 5)

Similarly, President Samaranch argued, 'Some International Federations had judicial problems, but this sanction can be changed - this was important to keep the unity of the federations inside the Olympic movement - all federations are very, very happy' (Magnay, 1999, February 6). Attempts to portray this compromise positively may not have been very effective though, for example, International Triathlon Union President Les McDonald claimed, 'The rest of the bloody world backed down from soccer and cycling' (Christie, 1999, February 5). Likewise, Australian Swimming President Terry Gathercole expressed his dissent:

> It diminishes the credibility of the IOC when a couple of sports can dictate to it. The IOC could kick them out, but I don't think that's going to happen, particularly not to soccer which is one of the higher profiles and most popular sports in the Games.
>
> (Smith, 1999b, February 5)

The IOC's compromise extended beyond the exceptional circumstances rule at the Lausanne Conference as it faced increasing challenges to its legitimacy based on the independence of a new organisation. For example, Dick Pound – who was a major lead in drafting the IOC proposals – stated:

> The comments on independence do not necessarily equate to divorce or complete separation from the Olympic movement. I do not think it is necessary to entirely separate from the Olympic movement to have the requisite degree of independence in this area.
>
> (McCullough, 1999, February 3)

He clearly makes the point that the IOC should not be excluded. He went on to later add that the IOC was 'ready to give governments a 50% role in the agency- and would expect the governments to contribute financially' (Wilson, 1999, February 3) demonstrating the IOC's bargaining position. The outcome in the declaration was that 'An independent International Anti-Doping Agency shall be established' (International Olympic Committee, 1999, p. 2). This declaration is evidently a compromise on the originally proposed OMADA headed by Samaranch and de Merode.

Again, the IOC portrayed the outcome of the conference as a success for anti-doping and the Olympic movement. President Samaranch typified this rhetoric: 'I believe sincerely that this anti-doping conference was a big victory for clean sport. This was a positive, open, democratic debate. As for any important decision, forward progress is never a straight path' ('Comments from final day', 1999, February 4). Not all parties were convinced though, for example, John Mendoza from the Australian Sports Drug Agency voiced his disappointment: 'This is a lost opportunity and a very disappointing preliminary outcome from the conference' (Connolly, 1999, February 4), and Mark Sisson, director of the Triathlon Anti-Doping Commission declared: 'The big winners here are the lawyers of the world' (Humphries, 1999, February 5). It appears, then, that not all stakeholders were convinced by the bargain struck between the IFs, governments and the IOC.

Finally, we argue that the IOC's compromise can be seen in the design it presented for WADA as the Executive Committee positions were split equally between the Olympic movement and government representatives. Pound commented on this arrangement: 'We've had six or seven meetings of our working group that involves the Olympic movement and public authorities. I think we have a very high degree of agreement on establishing the agency' ('IOC committed', 1999, September 14). The IOC relied on its financial contribution to justify its position; for example, from the outset Pound argued, 'The governments must be prepared to put their money and efforts where their mouths are. We're not going to entertain a situation where they come and tell us how we spend our money' (Casert, 1999, February 5). Given that the IOC was able to place Dick Pound as the inaugural president of WADA without an election and ensure half the Executive Committee were Olympic movement members with vested interest in the IOC's success, we argue that the new organisation may well have been considered an effective compromise for Samaranch. On the subject of being the new WADA President, Pound originally explained:

> I'm prepared to do it for a year or so to get it up and running. My knowledge of this field is very limited, but what I would bring is the ability to get it organized and started and to adopt the policies that we need to adopt.
> ('Dick Pound to head', 1999, November 8)

However, Pound remained in the position for eight years. Had he not left his post in IOC's marketing commission (Mackay, 2001, December 22), the IOC may have had greater influence.

In summary, the IOC's willingness to bargain when presented with legitimacy challenges appears to have been an effective strategy in the long run as it was able to retain a controlling stake in WADA and the regulation of anti-doping in Olympic sports. This compromise has since had major repercussions for the regulation of anti-doping under WADA.

Conclusion

The rationale of this case study was to discuss the legitimacy processes around the creation of WADA, to understand under what conditions WADA was legitimated and to give greater context and understanding to the remaining cases in this book. A number of significant factors, and in particular Samaranch's comments in El Mundo and the Salt Lake City scandal, undermined the perceived legitimacy of the IOC going into the Lausanne Conference. Consequently, the IOC's legitimacy was challenged on both pragmatic and moral criteria as it was judged that the IOC could not be trusted to regulate anti-doping efforts in sport. Interestingly, the governments who challenged the IOC had different initial motivations, but the consensus behind their combined challenges was enough to achieve institutional change. This chapter suggests that in WADA being validated and OMADA being dismissed, it was the judgement of the group of activist governments behind an independent agency that became dominant. In contrast, the IOC and the IFs which had previously controlled anti-doping, lost their autonomy and became subject to suppressor factors to conform with the newly validated organisation. This meant that new institutional pressures to conform with WADA as an institution originated at Lausanne. Throughout this period of legitimacy debate, the IOC ineffectively responded to criticisms and pressures. However, the IOC's attempts to compromise were more effective as it was able to maintain representation on WADA's Executive Committee, keep a controlling financial stake in the organisation and install an IOC member as inaugural WADA President.

The outcome of the legitimacy challenges faced by the IOC and its responses are that WADA was institutionalised in a state of weak validity (Haack & Sieweke, 2018). This means that WADA's legitimacy does not reflect widespread consensus in the field of anti-doping about the value of the organisation. The IOC was unable to effectively manage legitimacy challenges, so a small group of governments validated their judgements suppressing not only the IOC and IFs but also every other nation that competes at the Olympic Games regardless of their own propriety judgements. These findings are important for establishing the context for the following cases. The institutional change which led to the creation of WADA illustrates the clear difference between sources who wish to control their own anti-doping procedures (e.g., IFs) and those who support WADA (e.g., activist governments). These defined groups have gone on to contest the legitimacy of WADA throughout its existence as we will now explore in the case studies.

References

Ames, P. (1999, October 19). EU cautious on world anti-doping agency, plans talks with IOC. Retrieved from https://apnews.com/.

Australian Olympic chief claims drug code ineffective. (1999, September 8). The Associated Press. Retrieved from https://apnews.com/.

Canadian Olympic Association. (1998). [Revised Canadian position and recommendations on doping in sport], *British Olympic Association archive collection* (GB 2381 BOA/IOC/M/12/2). UK: University of East London Archives, December 16.

Casert, R. (1999, January 26). Out-of-competition doping tests imminent in soccer. *The Associated Press*. Retrieved from https://apnews.com/.

Casert, R. (1999, January 29). FIFA and IOC at center of world doping conference next week With Sports. The Associated Press. Retrieved from https://apnews.com/ .

Casert, R. (1999, February 1). IOC faces uphill battle to get all federations behind global drug package. *The Associated Press*. Retrieved from https://apnews.com/.

Casert, R. (1999, February 2). Samaranch calls for 'autonomous' anti-drug agency. *The Associated Press*. Retrieved from https://apnews.com/.

Casert, R. (1999, February 3). AP Photos XLAU101-8. *The Associated Press*. Retrieved from https://apnews.com/.

Casert, R. (1999, February 5). Politicians, once invited to IOC meet, aren't leaving. *The Associated Press*. Retrieved from https://apnews.com/.

Casini, L. (2009). Global hybrid public-private bodies: The World Anti-Doping Agency (WADA). *International Organizations Law Review*, 6(2), 421–446.

Christie, J. (1999, January 5). Drug row may mean end to Olympic soccer. *The Globe and Mail*. Retrieved from https://www.theglobeandmail.com/.

Christie, J. (1999a, February 4). U.S. slammed for drug policies: Lax American system no model for Olympic movement, critics say. *The Globe and Mail*. Retrieved from https://www.theglobeandmail.com/.

Christie, J. (1999b, February 4). Antidoping scheme fails athletes' test: Plan attacked because IOC to be involved in drug-fighting agency. *The Globe and Mail*. Retrieved from https://www.theglobeandmail.com/.

Christie, J. (1999, February 5). Rest of world dulls penalty claws. *The Globe and Mail*. Retrieved from https://www.theglobeandmail.com/.

Comments from final day of doping summit. (1999, February 4). The Associated Press. Retrieved from https://apnews.com/.

Connolly, S. (1999, February 4). Drug stance damages Olympic credibility. *The Associated Press*. Retrieved from https://apnews.com/.

Corder, M. (1999a, November 15). Governments begin discussing anti-doping initiatives. *The Associated Press*. Retrieved from https://apnews.com/.

Council of Europe. (1998). [Recommendations and resolutions adopted by the monitoring group], *British Olympic Association archive collection* (GB 2381 BOA/IOC/M/12/2). UK: University of East London Archives, November 5.

Dick Pound to head the new IOC world anti-doping agency. (1999, November 8). The Associated Press. Retrieved from https://apnews.com/.

Dimeo, P., & Møller, V. (2018). *The anti-doping crisis in sport: Causes, consequences, solutions*. London, UK: Routledge.

Dobbin, W. (1999, February 2). Drugs problem. *The Associated Press*. Retrieved from https://apnews.com/.

Doping summit impossible to meet goals. (1999, February 3). Xinhua News. Retrieved from http://www.xinhuanet.com/english/.

Edwards, B. (1999, February 3). Meeting in Lausanne, Switzerland, is hoping to develop a program to guard against athletes using illegal drugs to enhance performance. *National Public Radio*. Retrieved from https://www.npr.org/programs/morning-edition/?t=1541001171340.

EU ministers call for independent anti-doping agency. (1999, January 18). Xinhua News. Retrieved from http://www.xinhuanet.com/english/.

EU ministers insist on two-year doping ban. (1999, June 1). *The Associated Press.* Retrieved from https://apnews.com/.

EU to participate in new anti-doping body. (1999, November 2). *The Associated Press.* Retrieved from https://apnews.com/.

European Community sports minister. (1999, February 2). *The Associated Press.* Retrieved from https://apnews.com/.

Evagora, A. (1998, July 21). Drug scandal at Tour de France. *The Associated Press.* Retrieved from https://apnews.com/.

Executive Office of the White House. (1998, November 17). *[Recommendations of the White House Office of National Drug Control Policy]*, British Olympic Associati on archive collection (GB 2381 BOA/IOC/M/12/2), UK: University of East London Archives.

Ferstle, J. (2001). World conference on doping in sport. In W. Wilson & E. Derse (Eds.), *Doping in elite sport: The politics of drugs in the Olympic movement* (pp. 275–286). Champaign, IL: Human Kinetics.

Fish, M. (1999, January 26). IOC's troubles lead to concerns for White House's drug czar. *Atlanta Journal.* Retrieved from https://www.ajc.com/.

Fish, M. (1999, February 3). Many oppose IOC-run doping agency. *Atlanta Journal.* Retrieved from https://www.ajc.com/.

Fotheringham, W. (1998, November 28). Threat of Olympic exclusion to aid fight against drug use. *The Guardian.* Retrieved from https://www.theguardian.com/uk.

Franke, W.W., & Berendonk, B. (1997). Hormonal doping and androgenization of athletes: A secret program of the German Democratic Republic government. *Clinical Chemistry, 43*(7), 1262–1279.

Gleaves, J. (2011). Doped professionals and clean amateurs: Amateurism's influence on the modern philosophy of anti-doping. *Journal of Sport History, 38*(2), 237–254.

Gleaves, J., & Llewellyn, M. (2014). Sport, drugs and amateurism: Tracing the real cultural origins of anti-doping rules in international sport. *The International Journal of the History of Sport, 31*(8), 839–853.

Glynn, M.A., Watkiss, L., Raffaelli, R., & Blyler, M. (2012). When identity boundaries are breached: Examining the scandal of the 1998 Winter Olympics, *Proceedings of the New Frontiers in Management and Organizational Cognition Conference.* Maynooth: National University of Ireland.

Haack, P. & Sieweke, J. (2018). The Legitimacy of Inequality: Integrating the Perspectives of System Justification and Social Judgment. *Journal of Management Studies, 55*, 486–516. 10.1111/joms.12323.

Hanstad, D.V., Smith, A., & Waddington, I. (2008). The establishment of the World Anti-Doping Agency: A study of the management of organizational change and unplanned outcomes. *International Review for the Sociology of Sport, 43*(3), 227–249.

Hersh, P. (1999, March 15). IOC under heat to enact real reform. *The Calgary Herald,* Retrieved from https://calgaryherald.com/.

Houlihan, B. (2002). *Dying to win: Doping in sport and the development of anti-doping policy* (Vol. 996). Strasbourg, France: Council of Europe Publishing.

Humphries, T. (1999, February 5). New beginning for sport ends in old story. *The Irish Times.* Retrieved from https://www.irishtimes.com/.

Hunt, T.M. (2011). *Drug games: The International Olympic Committee and the politics of doping, 1960–2008.* Austin, TX: University of Texas Press.

Hunt, T.M., Dimeo, P., & Jedlicka, S.R. (2012). The historical roots of today's problems: A critical appraisal of the international anti-doping movement. *Performance Enhancement & Health, 1*(2), 55–60.

International Olympic Committee. (1999). Lausanne declaration on doping in sport. Lausanne, Switzerland.

IOC committed to drugs agency. (1999, September 14). The Associated Press. Retrieved from https://apnews.com/.

IOC official says federations could face punishment. (1998, November 13). The Associated Press. Retrieved from https://apnews.com/.

Longman, J. (1999, January 29). I.O.C. drug chief calls for shift in bans. *The New York Times.* Retrieved from https://www.nytimes.com/.

Mackay, D. (1999, February 5). Banks says no to new initiative to fight drugs. *The Guardian.* Retrieved from https://www.theguardian.com/uk.

Mackay, D. (2001, December 22). Olympic saviour abandons IOC. *The Guardian.* Retrieved from https://www.theguardian.com/uk.

Maennig, W. (2014). Inefficiency of the anti-doping system: Cost reduction proposals. *Substance Use & Misuse, 49*(9), 1201–1205.

Magnay, J. (1999, January 29). Cycling boss seeks rulings on legal drugs. *Sydney Morning Herald.* Retrieved from https://www.smh.com.au/.

Magnay, J. (1999, February 6). Dopes fail the test. *Sydney Morning Herald.* Retrieved from https://www.smh.com.au/.

Marshallsea, T. (1999, February 4). Drugs conference hit by soccer, cycling stance. *The Associated Press.* Retrieved from https://apnews.com/.

McCullough, E. (1999, February 2). Leadership. *The Associated Press.* Retrieved from https://apnews.com/.

McCullough, E. (1999, February 3). Olympic doping. *The Associated Press.* Retrieved from https://apnews.com/.

McCullough, E. (1999, February 4). Olympic doping blow. *The Associated Press.* Retrieved from https://apnews.com/.

McMillan, A. (1998, July 28). Ease drugs bans. Retrieved from https://www.dailytelegraph.com.au/.

Moore, M. (1998, July 29). Games drugs row boils over. *Sydney Morning Herald.* Retrieved from https://www.smh.com.au/.

Myers, M. (1998, September 14). Leading Olympic officials are against jailing athletes who take hard performance-enhancing drugs. *Agence France Presse.* Retrieved from https://www.afp.com/en.

Oliver, C. (1991). Strategic responses to institutional processes. *Academy of Management Review, 16*(1), 145–179.

Olympic delegate rebuffs Clinton advisor on drugs body. (1999, November 15). The Associated Press. Retrieved from https://apnews.com/.

Ritchie, I., & Jackson, G. (2014). Politics and 'shock': Reactionary anti-doping policy objectives in Canadian and international sport. *International Journal of Sport Policy and Politics, 6*(2), 195–212.

Rowbottom, M. (1999, February 3). Banks leads attack on 'sad, soured, sullied' IOC. Retrieved from https://www.independent.co.uk/.

Salvado, J. (1998, July 29). Doping in sport conference long overdue. *The Associated Press*. Retrieved from https://apnews.com/.

Salvado, J. (1998, July 30). Bigger role for law enforcement on sports drugs. *The Associated Press*. Retrieved from https://apnews.com/.

Salvado, J. (1999, August 5). IOC has ignored doping experts. *The Associated Press*. Retrieved from https://apnews.com/.

Samaranch calls for world conference on drugs. (1998, July 27). The Associated Press. Retrieved from https://apnews.com/.

Shipley, A. (1999, September 16). IOC drug plan is 'inadequate'. *The Washington Post*. Retrieved from https://www.washingtonpost.com/.

Smith, W. (1999a, February 5). Truth and consequence. *The Courier Mail*. Retrieved from https://www.couriermail.com.au/.

Smith, W. (1999b, February 5). IOC keeps drug cheat powers. *The Courier Mail*. Retrieved from https://www.couriermail.com.au/.

Stanaway, G. (1999, January 30). IOC plan for softer position on drugs. *The Courier Mail*. Retrieved from https://www.couriermail.com.au/.

Sydney summit plan to push hard line on drugs. (1999, February 6). *The Age*. Retrieved from https://www.theage.com.au/.

Thomson appalled over Samaranch remarks. (1998, July 28). The Associated Press. Retrieved from https://apnews.com/.

US criticized at Anti-Drug Conference. (1999, February 3). RTE. Retrieved from https://www.whitehouse.gov/.

U.S. track stars banned for drugs. (1998, July 28). The Associated Press. Retrieved from https://apnews.com/.

Waddington, I. (2016). Theorising unintended consequences of anti-doping policy. *Performance Enhancement & Health*, 4(3–4), 80–87.

Wagner, U., & Pedersen, K.M. (2014). The IOC and the doping issue—An institutional discursive approach to organizational identity construction. *Sport Management Review*, 17(2), 160–173.

Wilson, S. (1998, July 28). IOC denies softening stance on drugs. *The Associated Press*. Retrieved from https://apnews.com/.

Wilson, S. (1998, August 20). IOC proposes new anti-drug agency. *The Associated Press*. Retrieved from https://apnews.com/.

Wilson, S. (1999, February 1). Disputes emerge on eve of drug summit. *The Associated Press*. Retrieved from https://apnews.com/.

Wilson, S. (1999, February 2). Bribery scandal puts IOC under attack at opening of drug summit. *The Associated Press*. Retrieved from https://apnews.com/.

Wilson, S. (1999, September 23). IOC fights to defend its anti-drug policies. *The Associated Press*. Retrieved from https://apnews.com/.

Chapter 4

The whereabouts system

Given its disputatious existence, the whereabouts system is a critical topic in understanding how stakeholders view the legitimacy of the World Anti-Doping Agency (WADA). The whereabouts system is a policy that stipulates elite athletes must provide anti-doping authorities with a daily location at which they will be located for one hour so that testing can occur without warning. The previous chapter established that WADA was legitimated in a state of weak validation (i.e., there was a lack of consensus in the field of anti-doping). This chapter examines the whereabouts system and exposes how a central policy platform has invoked a need for WADA to respond to various legitimacy challenges. In doing so, we aim to demonstrate that WADA's legitimacy is vulnerable because of a lack of consensus in the field of anti-doping. Moreover, we suggest that WADA's response to the challenges created by the whereabouts system is characterised by coercion and resistance.

The primary tool in regulating performance-enhancing drug (PED) use in sport has historically been the biological testing of athletes to detect the presence of prohibited substances. Under WADA, the current anti-doping system still privileges testing as the cornerstone of regulation and has developed new complementary strategies, such as gathering information to test athletes when they are most likely to be doping. WADA has consistently supported the development of new and improved testing methods and technologies that are more sensitive to lower concentrations of prohibited substances. Despite the commitment to superior testing, WADA recognised that solely testing athletes at competitions was insufficient to detect doping because athletes could use prohibited substances prior to competition, reap the long-term training and performance benefits and then cease substance use far enough in advance of competition that it would not be detected whilst retaining the physiological benefits (Borry et al., 2018). As a result, the first World Anti-Doping Code (WADC) released in 2003 stipulated that all signatories would operate a whereabouts system to conduct unannounced out-of-competition (OOC) testing. The whereabouts system stipulates that 'athletes who have been included in a Registered Testing Pool by their International Federation and/or National Anti-Doping Organization shall provide whereabouts information in the manner specified in the International Standard for Testing and Investigations' (WADA, 2020, p. 9). This means that elite athletes chosen by an anti-doping organisation (e.g., a National Anti-Doping Organisation) must provide their location to anti-doping authorities for one hour per day every day, every three months. By doing so, athletes can be located by anti-doping organisations and tested without warning. The policy was designed to eradicate doping out of season.

Since its introduction, the whereabouts system has continually proven to be a controversial component of the anti-doping system. Among other issues, it has been associated with perceived infringements on athletes' human right for privacy, inequitable local implementation in different parts of the world and the relative ease with which OOC testing can be evaded (e.g., athletes hiding from anti-doping testers to avoid taking a test when they have recently taken a prohibited substance). Disparities in the implementation of the whereabouts policy have also led to distrust from athletes towards other nations perceived to be less stringent with anti-doping procedures (Bloodworth & McNamee, 2010; Hanstad & Loland, 2009; Henning & Dimeo, 2019). Studies have shown that athletes are uncertain about the whereabouts policy, and a significant proportion do not agree with the need to be available seven days a week and have had negative experiences because of the whereabouts system (Overbye & Wagner, 2014; Valkenburg, de Hon, & van Hilvoorde, 2014). This is substantiated by a synthesis of previous research addressing athlete perceptions of the anti-doping system under WADA, which signposts the obligation to submit whereabouts as one of four major issues of concern (Gleaves & Christiansen, 2019). As Waddington (2010) noted, 'What is clear is that the introduction of the whereabouts system has acted as a catalyst for a more general critique of the relationship between elite athletes and WADA and of the structure of decision-making processes within WADA' (p. 270).

The next section of this chapter explores the introduction of the whereabouts system. Three key periods of instability for the whereabouts system are identified that led to significant debate about the legitimacy of WADA. These are (1) the introduction of the whereabouts system in the first edition of the WADC; (2) the revised whereabouts system introduced in 2009; (3) British runner Mo Farah's missed OOC tests and links to athletics coach Alberto Salazar. Analysis of these events raises three key points for discussion. The first discussion point is Olympic independence, as stakeholders challenging the legitimacy of WADA shared the characteristic that they were not financially dependent upon Olympic participation. The second point is necessity as WADA argued that random OOC testing was crucial to the anti-doping system. Third, controlling obligation refers to WADA's responses to legitimacy challenges from athletes and organisations by reinforcing the organisations' authority.

The development of the whereabouts system

Before progressing to the analysis, in the following section, we outline how the three versions of the whereabouts system have developed and present analysis of previous academic research and criticisms of the policy. The first version of the WADC stipulated flexible requirements upon signatories to collect whereabouts information (i.e., the time and place at which they can be located on a given day) and required athletes to be available for testing five days a week (Halt, 2009). The result was a discordant system which placed varying levels of strictness upon athletes from different nations, thus negating the mission of WADA to harmonise regulations between signatories (Hanstad, Skille, & Loland, 2010). The whereabouts system was revised in the second version of the WADC and stipulated more precise rules to reduce variability in interpretation between signatories as well as increased amounts of data required from athletes. Furthermore, the second WADC specified that all athletes in a registered testing pool must pre-emptively provide their location for one hour per day, every day, for three months, to enable unannounced OOC testing (testing an athlete without warning). Athletes could commit a whereabouts violation if they failed to provide correct location information before the start of each quarter or if they were not present in a specified location and missed a test. Under this system, if an athlete committed a total of three whereabouts failures in an 18-month period, this constituted an anti-doping rule violation (ADRV) and the athlete received up to a two-year ban. The requirements of the whereabouts system were again revised in the third version of the WADC. The period in which three whereabouts failings constituted an ADRV was reduced from 18 to 12 months decreasing the risk of committing an ADRV (WADC, 2017, p. 21).

The significance of the whereabouts system for athletes is determined by the consequences of failing to provide correct information. The 1 January 2021 WADC update states: 'Any combination of three missed tests and/or filing failures, as defined in the International Standard for Results Management, within a 12-month period by an Athlete in a Registered Testing Pool' (WADC, 2020, p. 22) is considered an ADRV ranging from a minimum of one- to a maximum of two-year suspension depending on culpability and previous behaviour. The culpability of the athlete in failing to provide correct whereabouts information is determined by the perceived intent to deceive testers as stated in the WADC:

> The flexibility between two (2) years and one (1) year of Ineligibility in this Article is not available to Athletes where a pattern of last-minute whereabouts changes or other conduct raises a serious suspicion that the Athlete was trying to avoid being available for Testing.
>
> (WADC, 2020)

Given the potential seriousness of failing to provide whereabouts information and the perceived infringements on an athlete's human right to privacy in their personal and home life, the whereabouts system has met stern opposition from different stakeholders since its introduction (Halt, 2009; Waddington, 2010). For example, the International Federation of Association Football (FIFA) and the Union of European Football Associations (UEFA) both refused to impose whereabouts regulations on individual athletes within a team (FIFA, 2009). In addition, British athletes met directly with WADA to voice concerns (BBC, 2009), while 65 Belgian athletes challenged the requirements in the Belgian Council of State, the highest administrative court of Belgium (Alvad, 2009). The uneasy relationship between athletes and the whereabouts system has been a hallmark of the system's existence which is still subject to scrutiny from a human rights perspective.

Ethical commentary of the whereabouts system has been predominantly negative, raising questions about the justification of surveillance and potential infringements on an athlete's human rights (Halt, 2009; Hardie, 2014; Kreft, 2009; Møller, 2011; Waddington, 2010). Specifically, MacGregor, Griffith, Ruggiu and McNamee (2013) highlighted that the whereabouts system may be in violation of the 1998 European Human Rights Act. In 2011, a collective of French athlete unions brought a case to the European Court of Human Rights arguing that WADA's whereabouts system violated article 8 of the European Convention on Human Rights: the right to respect for private and family life. We agree that there is merit in the argument that athletes are subject to infringements on privacy not defensible in most other jobs, but the problem is whether the infringements on privacy outweigh the risks to health posed by doping. In 2018 the European Court of Human Rights ruled against the unions disputing the clauses MacGregor et al. cited as potential violations:

> To reduce or remove the obligations of which they complained would be capable of increasing the dangers of doping for their health and for that of the whole sports community, running counter to the European and international consensus on the need for unannounced testing.
>
> (European Court of Human Rights, 2018, p. 19)

Despite the criticisms of surveillance and privacy intrusions put forward by the athletes and scholars, the European Court of Human Rights decision suggested that the privacy arguments were legally indefensible as the potential dangers of doping were judged to outweigh any harm caused by surveillance.

The specific rules of the whereabouts system are still a subject of debate and conjecture 16 years after their introduction. For instance, in 2017, two English Premier League football teams were fined for failing to provide correct locations to drug testers (MacInnes, 2017). Although this did not provide evidence of wrongdoing, it rekindled debates about the whereabouts system because failure to provide correct information exemplified concerns about the potential to conceal doping. If an individual player provided a positive test for a prohibited substance, he or she could receive up to a four-year suspension. Opposingly, when an organisation provides incorrect whereabouts information, it could receive a financial penalty. Therefore, the worst-case scenario is that sport organisations provide incorrect whereabouts information to protect doping athletes.

The whereabouts system is also subject to debate because athletes can be sanctioned for inadvertent errors in data provision rather than an intention to 'cheat'. The potential for non-doping athletes to be sanctioned for filing errors challenges the legitimacy of the whereabouts system as a mechanism to protect athletes playing by the rules (Moston & Engelberg, 2019). Critics of the whereabouts system have pointed to the opportunity for athletes to avoid drug testing by providing vague whereabouts information in remote training environments, changing their location at the last minute, deliberately missing tests that they will not be able to pass and micro-dosing (taking substances in a small enough dosage to avoid detection but enough to accumulate performance enhancement) (Marty, Nicholson & Haas, 2015). Given the severe impositions on privacy the whereabouts system places on all athletes against the backdrop of these practical constraints, the whereabouts system remains a source of debate in anti-doping. The next section will outline the details of key events related to the whereabouts system that have challenged the legitimacy of WADA.

The whereabouts system: key periods of instability

Although there are numerous contentious incidents involving the whereabouts system, the following periods of instability (Bitektine & Haack, 2015) were chosen as they led to verbal (e.g., public criticism) and behavioural (e.g., refusal to implement policy) challenges that brought the policy and WADA's legitimacy into question (Deephouse, Bundy, Tost, & Suchman, 2017). Furthermore, these challenges elicited a direct response from WADA as the organisation sought to maintain its legitimacy symbolically (e.g., press release) or substantively (e.g., policy change) (Ashforth & Gibbs, 1990; Deephouse et al., 2017). For example, the US Anti-Doping Agency's (USADA) decision (in consultation with WADA) to drop the case against 100-m American sprinter Christian Coleman for three whereabouts failures in 2019, because the infringements were not all within a 12-month period, was a high-profile event. However, discussions following this decision did not present a legitimacy challenge, and in response WADA stated it would not contest USADA's decision. Likewise, Coleman's fourth career whereabouts failing in June 2020 was a high-profile event, but discussion did not involve WADA and instead focused on why Coleman had committed a fourth whereabouts failing. At the time of writing, Coleman's case is ongoing, and he is provisionally suspended. The reason the case has not led to legitimacy challenges is seemingly because Coleman admits to not being at the specified whereabouts location, and was instead shopping locally (Ingle, 2020).

The first period of instability we examine concerns the introduction of the whereabouts system in the first WADC in 2004. Prior to the first WADC, anti-doping was criticised for a lack of whereabouts information and OOC testing. Critics noted that anti-doping efforts were being undermined by athletes that trained in remote locations to avoid testers. Therefore, in the first edition of the WADC, whereabouts requirements were introduced to accommodate varying levels of resources that enabled signatories greater discretion to determine what information was required from athletes, when they were required for testing, what constituted a filing mistake and what punishment could be instigated (Dikic, Markovic, & McNamee, 2011; Hanstad et al., 2010). Following this, a period emerged where stakeholders such as FIFA, UEFA and a group of Belgian Sporting officials challenged the whereabouts system arguing that it unfairly impeded athlete privacy. Furthermore, in 2006 British 400-m sprinter Christine Ohuruogu was deemed by the British Olympic Association to have committed an anti-doping violation due to missing three OOC tests. At the time, the British whereabouts system was recognised as one of the strictest systems because if an athlete was not at his or her specified location, testers could not ring the athlete to notify that he or she was required for testing. Ohuruogu's subsequent suspension and the lack of sympathy from sporting officials led to legitimacy challenges for the whereabouts system as critics pointed to the unfairness of the system (Verroken, 2007). Consequently, in the second edition of the WADC, WADA sought to manage perceptions of its legitimacy by updating signatory requirements to ensure greater harmonisation.

The second period of instability occurred on January 1, 2009 when the second version of the WADC was introduced. The revised whereabouts system generated a large amount of public attention. The introduction of the revised system was arguably the most significant period in relation to the whereabouts system as it engaged a wide range of stakeholders who challenged WADA due to negative perceptions of the mandatory increased surveillance. Stakeholders that challenged the new WADC included FIFA, the Board of Control for Cricket in India (BCCI), a group of Belgian athletes, the European Court of Human Rights, numerous athletes from across Olympic sports, the World Tennis Association (WTA) and the Spanish Government. The verbal criticisms and refusal to implement the new rules varied in severity and longevity but involved a common negative judgement about the increased surveillance advocated in the second edition of the WADC.

The third period of instability began in June 2015 after the disclosure that Olympic 5,000-m and 10,000-m champion Mo Farah had missed two OOC tests in 12 months alongside accusations that his coach Alberto Salazar had committed ADRVs involving other athletes, which were later established in 2019 (but are subject to appeal at the time of writing). Missing two OOC tests is not evidence of any wrongdoing but the event raised discussion among stakeholders about the whereabouts system as they questioned the legitimacy of WADA's policy, thus forcing the organisation to respond. Having outlined the details of each period of instability, these periods will now be considered to examine how the legitimacy of WADA has been challenged and how WADA has responded.

The following discussion will focus on three key points: (1) Olympic independence, (2) necessity and (3) controlling obligation.

Olympic independence

Olympic independence captures how stakeholders that challenged WADA's legitimacy were characterised by their lack of dependence upon the IOC for funding. Football, cricket and tennis are all financially independent of the IOC as the Olympic Games are not their primary source of income. These sports are what Maennig (2014) terms *media sports*, where 'large television source figures lead to a strong willingness to pay for the sponsorship and/or television commercials by companies' (p. 1205). Independence from the IOC reduces the severity of suppressor factors (i.e., threat of reputational damage and potential gain from compliance) giving independent organisations more freedom to contest WADA's legitimacy. The Olympic Charter stipulates that to be recognised as an International Federation (IF) by the IOC, an IF must adopt the WADC (IOC, 2019). Challenges to the legitimacy of WADA came from FIFA, the BCCI, WTA and prominent athletes from within these sports who refused to abide by the whereabouts system because it was perceived as unworkable and intrusive. This group of organisations were characterised by arguments launched against WADA that the whereabouts system was a violation of an athlete's privacy rights and that it was not necessary for athletes in team sports to provide individual whereabouts information when they could be located with their club. The willingness of these stakeholders to challenge WADA and avoid their Olympic obligations suggests that the threat of Olympic expulsion was insufficient to stop them from expressing judgements about the legitimacy of the anti-doping policy.

Following the introduction of the first WADC, despite deliberate flexibility in how the whereabouts system could be implemented to allow for differences in resources and experience between signatories (Hanstad et al., 2010), sports organisations still contested the system. For example, in Australia, representatives of cricket, Australian rules football, rugby league and rugby union raised concerns about three missed tests constituting an ADRV (Masters, 2004, December 10). FIFA declared it would not be collecting whereabouts data (Warner, 2004, May 4). There is also the possibility that these organisations were concerned about allowing external regulation of their sport. These organisations, however, are not as dependent upon Olympic participation for commercial exposure. Therefore, the initial threat of expulsion for failing to comply with the WADC – which coerces other organisations to remain silent and not express their legitimacy judgements – does little to suppress their negative judgements. This dynamic can also be seen following the introduction of the second WADC.

The second WADC was subject to legitimacy challenges before it came into effect on January 1, 2009. The concerns raised prior to the WADC coming into effect suggest that the consultation process was enough to engage signatories in actively evaluating the revisions to the whereabouts system and voicing concerns. For example, in March 2008, FIFA President Sepp Blatter offered conditional acceptance of the revised WADC meaning it would not be implemented until FIFA was satisfied with the rules. He argued that it was not appropriate for footballers to provide individual information when they could be located with their team and declared that acceptance of the policy would be contingent upon the removal of the individual location stipulation ('Four more Years', 2008, March 1). Blatter's challenge was rooted at a moral level as he argued the invasion of privacy was not justifiable or necessary in football. Similarly, Scottish Players Football Association chief Fraser Wishart questioned the need for whereabouts in football: 'I can understand the whereabouts ruling for athletes, but not in football where every player has a place of work' (Campbell, 2008, November 16). Other sports have also challenged the system's appropriateness; in June 2008, Stuart Miller, ITF Anti-Doping Head, stated:

> Tennis is not like athletics in the sense that those taking part do not map out their training programme and the two or three events they are going to take part in at the start of the year. Tennis players take part in single-elimination competitions and if they get knocked out on day one of an event they'll simply move on to another one, go home or go on holiday. The most important thing from the point of view of the whereabouts provision is that they are not going to be where they said they would be and if you imagine all the players in our pool having to provide us with constantly updated information and us having to keep track of that, it's fair to say there are going to be significant problems going forward.
>
> (Nakrani, 2008, June 18)

Miller's comments are another example that, while an Olympic sport, tennis is not dependent upon it for survival. As such, Miller was able to challenge the legitimacy of WADA on behalf of the ITF with reduced fear of reputational or financial repercussions.

When the second WADC became active in January 2009, further challenges were issued. FIFA continued to challenge the whereabouts system's legitimacy on the belief that it was inappropriate for footballers. A joint announcement from FIFA and UEFA stated:

> The governing bodies of FIFA and UEFA formally reject the stance taken by WADA concerning the 'whereabouts' rule and, more specifically, the individual location of team sports' athletes. FIFA and UEFA wish to point out the fundamental differences between an individual athlete, who trains on his own, on the one hand, and a team sport's athlete, who is present at the stadium six days out of seven, and thus easy to locate, on the other hand. FIFA and UEFA therefore oppose the individual 'whereabouts' rule

and want to see it replaced by collective location rules, within the scope of
the team and within the stadium infrastructure.

(FIFA, 2009)

In this statement, FIFA argued for a different system in which OOC testing was
conducted in a manner that was suitable to football. FIFA's argument suggested
a shift in position as the need for OOC testing was not disputed; however, there
was a clear difference in judgements about violating an athlete's rights to
privacy in his or her personal life, including not disclosing his or her location.
FIFA's concerns were resolved in October 2009 when FIFA and WADA agreed
that only players who were coming back from injury or had previously been
sanctioned for an ADRV would need to provide whereabouts information. FIFA
would determine who should be in the testing pool to provide whereabouts
information based on high-risk athletes rather than elite athletes ('FIFA Doping
Deal', 2009, April 9). WADA President John Fahey presented this as intelligent
anti-doping strategy declaring: 'The important thing is to be smarter about what
you do with doping. It's about focusing on the people that are likely to be
cheating rather than simply doing blanket testing' ('WADA commit', 2009,
October 29). The agreement between FIFA and WADA demonstrated compromise, yet we argue that FIFA achieved the better outcome as its elite athletes
were not forced to provide whereabouts information.

The BCCI, responsible for Cricket in India, refused to agree to the whereabouts system following negative comments from senior players. In July 2009,
BCCI officials expressed their concerns:

> We understand the fears of the players and that's why we want to take a
> stock of the situation. Football doesn't adhere to WADA's out-of-contest
> testing, and there are several tennis players who have openly come out
> against this process. So there can be a debate on this issue.
>
> ('BCCI might back players', 2009, July 30)

The BCCI's statement reflected concerns from players about having to disclose
their whereabouts as they felt it violated their right to personal privacy and
created potential security risks if their whereabouts information was not kept
securely ('Accept WADA', 2009, July 5). The BCCI's statement also indicated
that the stance of FIFA acted as a cue to suggest that the BCCI and players were
not the only group holding a negative judgement. The cue from FIFA may have
encouraged the BCCI to challenge WADA. The challenge was at a moral level
as the BCCI officials and players had different beliefs to WADA about the right
to preserve privacy. The comments of BCCI President Shashank Manohar
clarified this position: 'Cricket should be WADA compliant. But the system of
testing was never discussed at the International Cricket Council. Our players are
ready to be tested but they say they are not in a position to give their whereabouts' (Dwivedi, 2009, August 2). A BCCI working committee defended its

position by reference to the Indian constitution arguing that human rights to privacy 'cannot be invaded' (Ali, 2009, August 2). Ratnakar Shetty, a senior BCCI official, used the same argument as football and tennis arguing that 'since the demands of cricketers are dissimilar from other sports, sooner or later a cricketer-specific code would be needed ... the requirements of cricketers are different' (Ali, 2009, August 31).

Given that at the time the BCCI was launching the lucrative Indian Premier League cricket tournament and was the largest financial contributor to the International Cricket Council (ICC), it occupied a significant position of power within the ICC and determining policy in cricket globally. The BCCI's concerns progressed to a fundamental challenge to the legitimacy of WADA as the BCCI argued: 'Why should we be subjected to Olympic regulations when we are not an Olympic sport? We would like to see the ICC set up its own drug-testing unit, and we hope that other countries will agree' (Briggs, 2009, October 6). Eventually the BCCI's challenge resulted in the whereabouts clause being dropped by the ICC ('ICC defers', 2009, October 8). By July 2010, the ICC had its own anti-doping policy with reduced whereabouts requirements so that players did not have to disclose their location when on holiday (Mukherjee, 2010, July 15).

The combination of the BCCI's influence in the ICC and the ICC's status as a non-Olympic sport provided the conditions for change as the ICC took control over anti-doping regulation away from WADA. Moreover, just as FIFA's challenge acted as a cue to the BCCI, the BCCI's challenge provided a cue to the Professional Footballers Association (PFA) in the United Kingdom. When asked why players were challenging the whereabouts system, PFA general secretary Simon Taylor referenced both the BCCI and FIFA:

> The whereabouts rule is suffering a slow death and it has definitely got to be revised. I am sure David Howman [WADA Director General] will defend it robustly, but it has now been kicked into touch by so many different countries and sports - Indian cricket and FIFA are not doing it so all the others should ask why they should too.
>
> ('Sport shorts', 2009, September 8)

We suggest that this challenge supports how suppressor factors, such as the threat of reputational or financial loss, appear to be determined by an organisation's context. By retaining financial independence from the IOC and not being dependent on exposure at the Olympic Games, the threat of expressing deviant opinions was reduced for these stakeholders.

Olympic independence is critical in understanding the legitimacy of WADA. Multi-level legitimacy theory predicts that a jolt should lessen suppressor factors allowing individuals and groups to express deviant legitimacy judgements (Bitektine & Haack, 2015). The evidence presented supports that evaluators are influenced by the size of the jolt and the severity of suppressor factors. For example, stakeholders with strong negative judgements of WADA's legitimacy and little to lose from expression may utilise every available opportunity to voice their judgement as was the case with FIFA. Whereas stakeholders that risk severe re-percussions for expressing a deviant opinion may require a more extreme jolt (e.g., organisational corruption) to challenge the consensus of legitimacy. In the case of the whereabouts system, the severity of suppressor factors appears to be linked to a sport's financial autonomy from the IOC and Olympic participation. We suggest that this explains the inability of WADA and the IOC to convince the big four major American sports (e.g., Major League Baseball, National Basketball Association, National Football League, National Hockey League) to become signatories to the WADC. The major American sports leagues operate as profit-maximising businesses with franchises. Consequently, they are financially secure outside of the Olympic movement, and there is no incentive for them to allow external regulation of their competitions.

Necessity

A common theme in WADA's responses to legitimacy challenges was an argument that OOC testing was essential to anti-doping efforts. WADA's arguments were based on the belief that if anti-doping is to be successful, the need for OOC testing should surpass any criticism. WADA took the position that without whereabouts information available to test athletes at random, every day of the year, OOC testing could not function effectively. For example, a Foundation Board meeting in November 2003 provides insights into WADA's view on the importance of OOC. Deputy director of Doping Control Policy and Development Rob Koehler supported the conclusion from a symposium on OOC testing which highlighted: 'With regard to the provision of whereabouts information, the conclusions had been that whereabouts information was of vital importance' (WADA, 2003). WADA's argument of necessity is also partly due to a lack of viable alternatives to replace random OOC testing. For ex-ample, after the second WADC became active, FIFA suggested that footballers should be entitled to an uninterrupted holiday without the stress of providing whereabouts information (Keating, 2009, May 11). Similarly, the BCCI argued that international cricket players should be entitled to a certain amount of uninterrupted holiday per year (Premachandran, 2009, August 12). In both cases, WADA suggested any breaks in OOC would undermine the entire system. WADA President John Fahey (2008–2013) maintained:

> One of the key principles of efficient doping control is the surprise effect and the possibility to test an athlete without advance notice on a 365-day basis. Alleging, as FIFA and UEFA do, that testing should only take place at training grounds and not during holiday periods, ignores the reality of doping in sport. Experience has demonstrated that athletes who cheat seize every opportunity to do so and dope when they believe they won't be tested.
>
> (Moore, 2009, March 26)

Fahey's emphasis on the utility of OOC testing is used to justify its necessity. WADA's defiance may be attributable to the reality that the difference in beliefs between WADA and its evaluators was insurmountable regarding the whereabouts system.

In 2009 the legitimacy of WADA was challenged as 65 Belgian athletes launched a legal challenge arguing that the whereabouts system violated their human rights, and in particular the right to privacy (Gibson, 2009, April 22). WADA was defiant when initially presented with the Belgian challenge. Their defence of the system explained: 'Because out-of-competition tests can be conducted without notice to athletes, they are one of the most powerful means of deterrence and detection of doping and are an important step in strengthening athlete and public confidence in doping-free sport' ('Anti-drug bosses', 2009, February 4). In the same period, an EU Sports Commission working group which investigated the legality of the whereabouts system regarding privacy laws determined that there were 'numerous issues that remain problematic' (Gibson, 2009, April 22). The Commission informed EU members that 'they must disregard the WADA drug code when it contradicts domestic law' (Magnay, 2009, April 23). In response, WADA President John Fahey expressed his disappointment:

> It contains some regrettable factual errors and could potentially undermine the fight against doping. WADA repeatedly offered to meet with the working party to provide more information and clarifications, but the European Commission, acting as the working party secretariat, regrettably turned down our requests. By challenging well-established and accepted anti-doping practices and offering no constructive solutions, the working party could potentially undermine the fight against doping in sport.
>
> (Gibson, 2009, April 22)

Spanish legislators presented a similar argument to the EU that gave athletes the right to refuse doping tests at night (Magnay, 2009, April 23). The EU Commission and Spanish legislators disputed the underpinning values of the whereabouts system (i.e., OOC testing is more important than surveillance infringements) and in doing so could have made WADA redundant as the chief regulator of anti-doping. If judicial organisations, such as the EU, have legal authority to overrule policies created by WADA, the legitimacy of the anti-doping system is subject to the decisions of national and international courts. WADA's approach to the legal challenges presented by the Belgian Court case and EU working group was again one of defiance. In the first instance, WADA advocated the merits of the system. It then adopted a more aggressive stance towards the findings of the EU Working Group by attacking the source of the challenge. Threatened with the possibility of losing control over the whereabouts system, WADA sought to discredit the judgements advocated by the EU, which served as a strong cue to other stakeholders due to its regulatory authority. When it was deemed that the whereabouts system violated European data laws, EU data experts made it clear: 'WADA was left in no doubt that the funding it receives from governments was at risk if it continued to fight existing data-protection laws' (Scott, 2009, May 12) indicating an uneasy tension between the legitimacy of WADA and European courts.

The same argument was visible from WADA six years later following the 2015 high-profile leak of Mo Farah missing two OOC tests before his success at the 2012 London Olympic Games (Lawton, 2015, June 18). In response to comments about Mo Farah, WADA President Sir Craig Reedie asserted:

> The reality is the whereabouts system is the best way to keep the sport clean. We need be able to do surprise, unannounced, out-of-competition testing. We realise that people can be careless or make mistakes and, in a sense, that has been recognised. Previously, it would have been a rule violation if an athlete clocked up three missed tests in 18 months, whereas now there has to be three missed tests in 12 months.
>
> (Reedie, 2015, July 9)

WADA's defiant response maintained its immutable posture to challenges based around privacy rights but revealed the steps it had taken to improve the whereabouts system. In other instances, WADA dismissed challenges to the legitimacy of the whereabouts system based on the assumption that no other feasible alternative exists. For example, in response to numerous criticisms from athletes, WADA Director General David Howman (2003–2016) argued on behalf of the Executive Committee: 'We haven't heard a suggestion of anything better ... This consultation took 18 months to two years before it was settled, so people had plenty of time to think of a better idea but we didn't hear one' ('WADA defends system', 2009, February 8).

With advances in technology and the accuracy of geolocational information, some athletes have suggested that they would rather be tracked than forced to go through the cumbersome process of providing whereabouts information for a three-month period. American hurdler Lolo Jones expressed her feelings towards tracking, 'I don't care if they have to put GPS on me 24/7. If that's what it takes to keep the sport clean, by all means I'm for it' (Clarey, 2009, March 2). Similarly, Canadian triathlete Simon Whitfield said: 'I'll start tomorrow if only to not have to fill out this insane form. I have nothing whatsoever to hide. You can track my whereabouts via GPS to your heart's content' (Clarey, 2009, March 2). WADA dismissed suggestions of scrapping the whereabouts system for a geolocational technological approach, and WADA's ethics committee noted its confidence in the current system:

> Subjecting athletes to reporting their whereabouts is already an exceptional measure that can only be legitimised by its aim (anti-doping) and means (its voluntary character). With regard to the latter, athletes may withdraw from surveillance if they quit elite sport, they are aware of the sanctions and the system is transparent.
>
> (Borry et al., 2018, p. 2)

Borry et al. (2018) went further stressing: 'However, it should be considered that various athletes already perceive the current whereabouts system as privacy infringing and that adding geolocalisation would only increase this feeling. Moreover, only a minority of athletes support such devices' (p. 3). These comments from WADA's ethics panel reaffirmed the organisation's belief of the whereabouts system's necessity because of its aim to achieve doping-free sport.

In summary, like Waddington's (2010) analysis, our analysis suggests that WADA has been defiant in response to legitimacy challenges related to the whereabouts system. However, we argue that this defiance can be explained by a divergence in values between WADA and its sources that is so large that it cannot be solved.

Controlling obligation

Building on Olympic independence and necessity, the following section presents the final discussion point from our analysis of the whereabouts system's legitimacy, controlling obligation. It is evident in the periods of instability that WADA has tried to manipulate legitimacy challenges (Oliver, 1991) by exerting its authority over challengers at two levels: (1) athletes and (2) WADC signatories. Regarding athletes, WADA used its legal dominance to make the point that athletes were free to either withdraw from competitive sport or they must accept the whereabouts system. But as Waddington (2010) discussed, athletes do not have this choice having usually dedicated their whole life to the pursuit of a professional sporting career. WADA used its position of authority over athletes to demand that athletes agree to the WADC. The second level of control was aimed at dissenting signatories. WADA declared that any anti-doping or sporting organisation that did not comply with the whereabouts system risked being labelled non-compliant and faced the potential of Olympic exclusion.

At the athlete level, there is a clear discourse from WADA and Olympic officials that if athletes want clean sport, they must make sacrifices, and if they are unwilling to make concessions, they do not need to participate in elite sport. Following the introduction of the first WADC (effective from January 1, 2004) and Christine Ohuruogu's whereabouts ADRV, WADA President Dick Pound (2000–2007) observed: 'Get organised. You know as a professional athlete that doping controls are a very important part of making your sport fair and it's your responsibility to tell your federation where you are, and to be where you say you're going to be' (Rowbottom, 2006, August 9). Jacques Rogge, former President of the IOC (2001–2013), lent further support to the whereabouts system following challenges to the second WADC (effective from January 1, 2009): 'Sports today has to pay a price for suspicion. The best way to alleviate the suspicion is allow for out-of-competition testing' (Clarey, 2009, March 2). We argue that this suggests that there is an obligation on the athletes to pay a price if they want to continue competing. Likewise, the comments of David Howman, Director General of WADA, highlighted the same obligations on athletes:

I don't feel sorry for these athletes because this is what life has come to for all of us. The rest of us must go through security at the airport and have our movements monitored. All because a small group of people ruined it for everyone else.

(Macur, 2009, March 23)

WADA's Executive Committee justified this approach by arguing that most stakeholders supported the whereabouts system (WADA, 2010, May 8). WADA's position suggested that many athletes accept the need for whereabouts but still experienced issues with its implementation (Overbye & Wagner, 2014).

The power relationship between athletes and WADA is unequally distributed, and this is crucial to understanding WADA's control over athletes. As Waddington (2010) noted, 'Athletes are subject to a system of surveillance and control which was introduced without their consent, by a body on which they have no proper representation' (p. 270). Whether professional athletes truly have a choice is contentious. Kreft (2009) argued that athletes do not opt into the whereabouts system because, as WADA suggested, they can choose to compete by the rules or quit. Møller (2011) argued that under the European Social Charter the whereabouts system was indefensible as similar levels of surveillance are not imposed in other occupations. Considering that the vast majority of athletes have dedicated their lives to achieving elite status making financial, educational and emotional sacrifices to do so (Waddington, 2010), very few have the 'simple' choice of leaving professional and elite sport to begin another career. From this perspective, WADA has dominance over individual athletes who hold negative judgements about the whereabouts system. The dependence of athletes on their sporting career and the need to submit to anti-doping regulations created a strong suppressor factor discouraging negative judgements of WADA.

The second level of controlling obligation focuses on WADA's response to legitimacy challenges from stakeholders at an organisational level. Following the implementation of the first WADC, certain sport organisations such as FIFA and the Australian Football League challenged the legitimacy of the whereabouts system. In Australia there was a negative judgement about the whereabouts rules (Masters, 2004, December 10). However, every Australian sport eventually signed due to the risk of losing financial support from the government. WADA was able to coerce compliance through its relationship with national governments. As Australian journalist Roy Masters noted:

An agreement reached between WADA and governments throughout the world obligates every signatory to cease funding to any sporting organisation that does not abide by the accord. The AFL [Australian Football League], the ARL [Australian Rugby League] and Cricket Australia have been set a deadline of June 30 to sign the WADA accord or lose all federal government funding.

(Masters, 2005, May 20)

Rather than attempt to answer their concerns, WADA used the possibility of losing financial support from the government as a mechanism to dominate sports organisations. It was not just the fear of financial loss that motivated organisations to comply. The need to be WADA compliant to achieve Olympic status served as a mechanism for WADA to leverage control over organisations challenging its legitimacy. For example:

> The ARU [Australian Rugby Union] has signed the WADA accord, despite the traditional dependence of footballers on GCS (glucocorticosteroids). It is understood rugby union's wish to be included on the Olympic program after the Beijing Olympics was a motivating factor in pledging support for the WADA list.
>
> (Masters, 2005, May 20)

We suggest that WADA's ability to prevent access to financial support and Olympic participation allowed it to establish the implementation of the first WADC despite negative judgements of the whereabouts system. Moreover, suppressor factors were evident in challenges to WADA such as those expressed by lawyer Bruce Collins on behalf of Cricket Australia in relation to the first WADC. Collins was sceptical of the appropriateness of the WADC to cricket. However, his statement noted: 'We also don't want to appear different to other sports' (Sygall, 2005, December 18), indicating that Cricket Australia recognised that failing to comply with the WADC could lead to reputational damage. We argue that as more evaluators with negative judgements complied with WADA due to suppressor factors, validity cues were reinforced and encouraged other sporting organisations to comply with the code and the rules of the whereabouts system.

Controlling obligation is seen with the introduction of the second WADC. Following FIFA's protests, David Howman, WADA Director General, declared: 'We would expect FIFA to co-operate. FIFA is now a WADA coded client' (Slot, 2008, February 29). There was a clear expectation in this statement that signatories should conform to the WADC. Similarly, WADA responded to FIFA by highlighting that by being non-compliant, FIFA risked being removed from the Olympic Games ('Nel retires', 2009, March 26). WADA took the same approach towards the BCCI as it sought to control the challengers through the Indian Government. However, the BCCI does not receive funding from the Indian Government and was not attempting to participate at the Olympic Games. Therefore, WADA had little power with which to coerce the BCCI. In both situations a compromise was ultimately forced. In FIFA's case, whereabouts requirements went ahead, but injured players and previous dopers were selected rather than elite players. The BCCI achieved a similar compromise as players were not required to disclose personal information as team location was deemed to be sufficient (Ali, 2011, February 12). In both instances WADA made it clear that no compromise had been made. In regard to FIFA, WADA President John

Fahey said: 'The Code was accepted, and I might add unanimously, with those whereabouts requirements, and nothing has changed as far as we are concerned, we haven't made any concessions' (Keating, 2009, May 11). Similarly, Director General David Howman stated in relation to the BCCI: 'There has been no change to WADA's international standard for testing' (Ali, 2011, February 12).

The notion that WADA can control athletes and signatories through access to Olympic participation raises issues in relation to the management of anti-doping. Firstly, despite increasing athlete representation at WADA, anti-doping rules are determined in a way that gives athletes very little influence and even less ability to challenge regulations. At the signatory level, coerced compliance from organisations rather than perceived legitimacy is associated with non-compliance when signatories are not monitored (Hurd, 1999). We suggest that WADA's reliance on coercing compliance by threatening to remove access to Olympic sport explains the lack of behavioural support. Rather than responding to challenges in a way that may encourage signatories to positively judge the legitimacy of the whereabouts system, WADA has manipulated legitimacy judgements. Signatories may therefore maintain negative judgements that are suppressed and, in the absence of effective compliance monitoring by WADA, may result in lacklustre policy implementation.

Conclusion

This chapter addressed the legitimacy challenges WADA has faced due to the whereabouts system and how the organisation has responded. We have argued there are two primary contributions to understanding the legitimacy of WADA. Firstly, the legitimacy of WADA was challenged by sources that judged the whereabouts system to violate athlete privacy rights or questioned its suitability for certain sports. These challenges were lodged predominantly by sport organisations that were characterised by their independence from the IOC and the Olympic Games (e.g., FIFA, ITF, BCCI). Although some of these organisations are recognised by the IOC, none of them are primarily dependent on exposure in the Olympic Games to generate financial profits.

Secondly, WADA responded to legitimacy challenges through defiance and manipulative control via access to Olympic competition. WADA argued that the whereabouts system was necessary for effective OOC testing despite the infringements on the privacy rights of athletes and that sources should accept it or risk Olympic exclusion. These responses have served WADA well, as the whereabouts system has not been substantially revised since the second WADC. Furthermore, notwithstanding the problem of sophisticated doping programmes such as micro-dosing, athletes changing their whereabouts at the last minute and training in remote places to avoid testing, there is a lack of feasible alternatives. Despite WADA's unwillingness to compromise on the need for a whereabouts system, improving the process of providing whereabouts information for athletes has been a regular concern of the Executive Board. An example of this is the creation of a mobile app in 2013 to improve flexibility for athletes. However, the control wielded over signatories to stop challenges may have failed to change signatories' perceptions of legitimacy. The lack of consensus in the field about the legitimacy of WADA's whereabouts system demonstrates the organisation's vulnerability. We suggest that this vulnerability begins to explain WADA's lack of effectiveness, as the organisation must coerce support. In coercing support, signatories to the WADC may not support the organisation when they are not rigorously monitored for compliance.

In the next chapter, we analyse how the case of Lance Armstrong challenged the legitimacy of WADA and how the organisation responded. Armstrong's case demonstrated both the susceptibility of testing to subterfuge and WADA's increasing recognition of the utility of an intelligence and investigations strategy. In analysing Armstrong's case, we extend our argument to suggest that WADA is able to reinterpret organisational deficiencies to manage its legitimacy. The ability of WADA to manipulate legitimacy challenges consequently has significant implications for the anti-doping system.

References

Accept WADA clause, says OCA chief to India. (2009, July 5). Right Vision News. Retrieved from http://rightvision.com.pk/.

Ali, Q.M. (2009, August 2). Dope trick. Mail Today. Retrieved from https://www.indiatoday.in/mail-today.

Ali, Q.M. (2009, August 31). BCCI could come out with its own dope code. Mail Today. Retrieved from https://www.indiatoday.in/mail-today.

Ali, Q.M. (2011, February 12). Indian cricketers test negative for doping. Mail Today. Retrieved from https://www.indiatoday.in/mail-today.

Alvad, S. (2009). Whereabouts rule causes controversy. Retrieved from http://www.playthegame.org/news/news-articles/2009/whereabouts-rule-causes-controversy/.

Anti-drug bosses defend new rules. (2009, February 4). Daily Post. Retrieved from https://www.dailypost.co.uk/.

Ashforth, B.E., & Gibbs, B.W. (1990). The Double-Edge of Organizational Legitimation. Organization Science, 1, 177–194. 10.1287/orsc.1.2.177.

BBC. (2009). Athletes air issues over testing. The BBC. Retrieved from http://news.bbc.co.uk/sport1/hi/front_page/7892590.stm.

BCCI might back players in battle against WADA rules. (2009, July 30). Indian Express. Retrieved from https://indianexpress.com/.

Bitektine, A., & Haack, P. (2015). The 'macro' and the 'micro' of legitimacy: Toward a multilevel theory of the legitimacy process. Academy of Management Review, 40(1), 49–75.

Bloodworth, A., & McNamee, M. (2010). Clean Olympians? Doping and anti-doping: The views of talented young British athletes. International Journal of Drug Policy, 21(4), 276–282.

Borry, P., Caulfield, T., Estivill, X., Loland, S., McNamee, M., & Knoppers, B.M. (2018). Geolocalisation of athletes for out-of-competition drug testing: Ethical considerations.

Position statement by the WADA Ethics Panel. *British Journal of Sports Medicine*. 52(7), 456–459.

Briggs, S. (2009, October 6). India plea for ICC support as they stay defiant over drug tests. *The Daily Telegraph*. Retrieved from https://www.telegraph.co.uk/.

Campbell A. (2008, November 16). Drug test plans are 'overkill', says Wishart. *Sunday Herald*. Retrieved from https://www.heraldscotland.com/.

Clarey, C. (2009, March 2). Again, athletes are put to the test, but this time to prove they're clean. *The New York Times*. Retrieved from https://www.nytimes.com/.

Deephouse, D.L., Bundy, J., Tost, L.P., & Suchman, M.C. (2017). Organizational Legitimacy: Six Key Questions, *The SAGE Handbook of Organizational Institutionalism* (pp. 27–52). 10.4135/9781446280669.n2.

Dikic, N., Markovic, S.S., & McNamee, M. (2011). On the efficacy of WADA's whereabouts policy: Between filing failures and missed tests. *Deutsche Zeitschrift für Sportmedizin Jahrgang*, 62(10), 324–328.

Dwivedi, S. (2009, August 2). Board stands by the players. *Indian Express*. Retrieved from https://indianexpress.com/.

European Court of Human Rights. (2018). Information Note 214. *Case-law of the European Court of Human Rights*. Retrieved from https://www.echr.coe.int/Documents/CLIN_2018_01_214_ENG.pdf.

FIFA. (2009). *FIFA and UEFA reject WADA 'whereabouts' rule*. Retrieved from https://www.fifa.com/development/news/y=2009/m=3/news=fifa-and-uefa-reject-wada-whereabouts-rule-1040455.html.

FIFA doping deal. (2009, April 9). *The Times*. Retrieved from https://www.thetimes.co.uk/.

Four more years for Mascherano. (2009, March 1). *The Irish Times*. Retrieved from https://www.irishtimes.com/.

Gibson, O. (2009, April 22). EU puts WADA's 'whereabouts' rule in doubt. *The Guardian*. Retrieved from https://www.theguardian.com/uk.

Gleaves, J., & Christiansen, A.V. (2019). Athletes' perspectives on WADA and the code: A review and analysis. *International Journal of Sport Policy and Politics*, 11(2), 341–353.

Halt, J. (2009). Where is the privacy in WADA's whereabouts rule. *Marquee Sports Law Review*, 20, 267.

Hanstad, D.V., & Loland, S. (2009). Elite athletes' duty to provide information on their whereabouts: Justifiable anti-doping work or an indefensible surveillance regime? *European Journal of Sport Science*, 9(1), 3–10.

Hanstad, D.V., Skille, E.Å., & Loland, S. (2010). Harmonization of anti-doping work: myth or reality? *Sport in Society*, 13(3), 418–430.

Hardie, M. (2014). Making visible the invisible act of doping. *International Journal for the Semiotics of Law-Revue*, 27(1), 85–119.

Henning, A., & Dimeo, P. (2019). Perceptions of legitimacy, attitudes and buy-in among athlete groups: A cross-national qualitative investigation providing practical solutions. *The World Anti-Doping Agency*. Retrieved from https://www.wada-ama.org/en/resources/social-science/.

Hurd, I. (1999). Legitimacy and authority in international politics. *International Organization*, 53(2), 379–408.

ICC defers WADA's 'whereabouts' clause. (2009, October 8). *Mail Today*. Retrieved from https://www.indiatoday.in/mail-today.

Ingle, S. (2020). Christian Coleman defends himself after missing drugs test. *The Irish Times*. Retrieved from https://www.irishtimes.com/.

IOC. (2019). The Olympic Charter. Retrieved from https://stillmed.olympic.org/.

Keating, S. (2009, May 11). No doping concessions for FIFA. *Yukon News*. Retrieved from https://www.yukon-news.com/.

Kreft, L. (2009). The elite athlete – in a state of exception? *Sport, Ethics and Philosophy*, 3(1), 3–18.

Lawton, M. (2015, June 18). Farah missed 2 drug tests. *The Daily Mail*. Retrieved from https://www.dailymail.co.uk/home/index.html.

MacGregor, O., Griffith, R., Ruggiu, D., & McNamee, M. (2013). Anti-doping, purported rights to privacy and WADA's whereabouts requirements: A legal analysis. *FairPlay, Revista de Filosofia, Ética y Derecho del Deporte*, 1(2), 13–38.

MacInnes. P. (2017). FA's increased drug testing to focus on Premier League players. *The Guardian*. Retrieved from https://www.theguardian.com/football/2017/jul/31/drug-testing-fa-premier-league-players.

Macur, J. (2009, March 23). Rule requiring drug testers to know athletes' whereabouts draws protest. *The New York Times*. Retrieved from https://www.nytimes.com/.

Maennig, W. (2014). Inefficiency of the anti-doping system: Cost reduction proposals. *Substance Use & Misuse*, 49(9), 1201–1205.

Magnay, J. (2009, April 23). Spain, EU challenge legality of drug tests. *Sydney Morning Herald*. Retrieved from https://www.smh.com.au/.

Marty, D., Nicholson, P. , & Haas, U. (2015). Cycling independent reform commission: Report to the president of the Union Cycliste Internationale. Zurich, Switzerland.

Masters, R. (2004, December 10). Drugs chiefs hold secret powwow over latest trends. *Sydney Morning Herald*. Retrieved from https://www.smh.com.au/.

Masters, R. (2005, May 20). Ban on cortisone a giant headache for AOC. *Sydney Morning Herald*. Retrieved from https://www.smh.com.au/.

Møller, V. (2011). One step too far – about WADA's whereabouts rule. *International Journal of Sport Policy and Politics*, 3(2), 177–190.

Moore, B. (2009, March 26). Football's arguments against the new doping rule do not stand up to scrutiny. *The Daily Telegraph*. Retrieved from https://www.telegraph.co.uk/.

Moston, S., & Engelberg, T. (2019). And justice for all? How anti-doping responds to 'innocent mistakes'. *International Journal of Sport Policy and Politics*, 11(2), 261–274.

Mukherjee, S. (2010, July 15). ICC snubs WADA, adopts own code. *The Times of India*. Retrieved from https://timesofindia.indiatimes.com/.

Nakrani, S. (2008, June 18). New drugs policy unworkable, says federation. *The Guardian*. Retrieved from https://www.theguardian.com/uk.

Nel retires from international cricket. (2009, March 26). *Independent Online*. Retrieved from https://www.iol.co.za/pretoria-news.

Oliver, C. (1991). Strategic responses to institutional processes. *Academy of Management Review*, 16(1), 145–179.

Overbye, M., & Wagner, U. (2014). Experiences, attitudes and trust: An inquiry into elite athletes' perception of the whereabouts reporting system. *International Journal of Sport Policy and Politics*, 6(3), 407–428.

Premachandran, D. (2009, August 12). Indian cricket not playing a straight bat with WADA. *The Guardian*. Retrieved from https://www.theguardian.com/.

Reedie, C. (2015, July 9). Our rules are strong enough to stop the dopers cheating. *The Independent*. Retrieved from https://www.independent.co.uk/.

Rowbottom, M. (2006, August 8). Ohuruogu may not be alone in missing tests. *The Independent*. Retrieved from https://www.independent.co.uk/.

Scott, M. (2009, May 12). Threat forced WADA 'whereabouts' climbdown. *The Guardian*. Retrieved from https://www.theguardian.com/uk.

Slot, O. (2008, February 29). FIFA under pressure to toe line over new testing procedures. *The Times*. Retrieved from https://www.thetimes.co.uk/.

Sport shorts. (2009, September 8). *Irish News*. Retrieved from https://www.irishnews.com/.

Sygall, D. (2005, December 18). Fear over hard line on drugs. *Sydney Morning Herald*. Retrieved from https://www.smh.com.au/.

Valkenburg, D., de Hon, O., & van Hilvoorde, I. (2014). Doping control, providing whereabouts and the importance of privacy for elite athletes. *International Journal of Drug Policy, 25*(2), 212–218.

Verroken, M. (2007). Why I am delighted Ohuruogu stormed back to win gold. *The Times*. Retrieved from https://www.thetimes.co.uk/.

WADA. (2003). Minutes of the WADA Foundation Board Meeting November 2003. Retrieved from https://www.wada-ama.org/.

WADA. (2010). Minutes of the WADA Executive Committee Meeting 8 May 2010. Retrieved from https://www.wada-ama.org/.

WADA. (2020). International standard for testing and investigations. Retrieved from https://www.wada-ama.org.

WADA commit to creating new anti-doping program for top-level soccer players. (2009, October 29). *The Star*. Retrieved from https://www.thestar.com/?redirect=true.

WADA defends system. (2009, February 8). *The Telegraph*. Retrieved from https://www.telegraph.co.uk/.

WADC. (2017). World Anti-Doping Code 2015 with 2018 amendments. https://www.wada-ama.org/sites/default/files/resources/files/wada_anti-doping_code_2018_english_final.pdf.

WADC. (2020). World Anti-Doping Code 2021. https://www.wada-ama.org/sites/default/files/resources/files/wada_anti-doping_code_2018_english_final.pdf.

Waddington, I. (2010). Surveillance and control in sport: A sociologist looks at the WADA whereabouts system. *International Journal of Sport Policy, 2*(3), 255–274.

Warner, A. (2004, May 4). FIFA's bid to reduce length of penalty for drugs. *The Evening Standard*. Retrieved from https://www.standard.co.uk/.

Chapter 5

Lance Armstrong and the Union Cycliste Internationale

Lance Armstrong was once viewed as the most successful road racing cyclist ever, winning the Tour de France seven times between 1999 and 2005, before retiring. This achievement was made more remarkable given that he was diagnosed with testicular cancer that had spread to his brain, lungs and abdomen at the age of 25. Armstrong subsequently recovered and went on to create the Livestrong Foundation, a charity focused on cancer patients and survivors, in addition to his cycling exploits. The combination of Armstrong's cycling dominance, philanthropic work and story of survival transformed him into a global icon, which afforded him commercial and sponsorship opportunities with major brands such as Nike and Oakley (Hambrick, Frederick, & Sanderson, 2015).

Despite his success, accusations of doping marred Armstrong's career, yet no allegations were upheld during his cycling career. In 2010, former teammate Floyd Landis, who was already serving a ban for an anti-doping rule violation (ADRV), turned whistle-blower alleging that Armstrong had doped throughout his career as well as organising and coercing teammates to dope as well. The information led to an investigation by the US Justice Department which closed the inquiry unsuccessfully in 2012, but the testimonies gained under oath were used to press charges of non-analytical ADRVs (i.e., evidence of doping violations from methods other than testing) by the United States Anti-Doping Agency (USADA, 2012). In January 2013, Armstrong confessed to a career of organised systematic doping, which included collusion with the governing body of cycling, the Union Cycliste Internationale (UCI). In the preceding chapters, we have established that WADA's creation as an institution rested on a low level of consensus which, in turn, presented issues for its ongoing legitimacy. This chapter focuses on how the behaviour of former professional cyclist Lance Armstrong and the UCI executive body challenged the legitimacy of WADA and how the organisation responded.

The combination of Armstrong's high profile and position to many as a hero meant his case generated massive media attention globally (Hambrick et al., 2015). The revelation of UCI collusion, the realisation that athlete testing had been subverted for years and the involvement of a federal agency in an anti-doping investigation meant that Armstrong's case challenged the legitimacy of

WADA and forced a response. Armstrong's case raised concerns about the efficacy of anti-doping testing, as with the help of the UCI, the cyclist was able to successfully subvert the system. In response to the challenges raised, not only did WADA attack its challengers rather than address the issues raised, it also reinterpreted the success of the non-analytical approach used to catch Armstrong as justification for further powers in the WADC.

The following section provides an overview of the numerous accusations of doping throughout Armstrong's career, supported by commentary from previous academic research exemplifying why his case was so threatening to WADA's legitimacy. Next, we identify the key periods of instability in Armstrong's career that led to WADA's legitimacy being challenged, before presenting the three themes of the analysis describing the challenges WADA faced and its legitimacy strategy: (1) victimisation, (2) attacking the source and (3) reinterpreting testing inefficiencies. Victimisation draws together examples of how both Armstrong and the UCI positioned themselves as being unfairly targeted by WADA and used this position to question the anti-doping system. Accordingly, the next point 'attacking the source' explains how WADA attempted to discredit Armstrong and the UCI to undermine their criticisms. Lastly, reinterpreting testing inefficiencies is the second part of WADA's response as it used the success of the investigation into Armstrong to gain further regulatory powers.

The impact of Armstrong on anti-doping

Having been absent from the 1998 Tour de France and the Festina scandal due to his cancer treatment and convalescence, Armstrong's first Tour win in 1999 was seen as a fresh start for the tour organisers and the sport of cycling. However, evidence emerged in 2004 that Armstrong had received a backdated TUE (therapeutic use exemption – a medical certificate to use a prohibited substance with potentially performance enhancing effects for medicinal purposes) to cover a positive corticosteroid test result from the 1999 tour. The claims were later dismissed after Armstrong sued for libel. In 2005, French newspaper L'Équipe reported that retrospective testing of Armstrong's urine samples from the 1999 Tour, as part of a scientific experiment, had returned positive results for the prohibited substance erythropoietin (EPO). This spurred the UCI to launch an investigation into the handling of the samples by the French anti-doping laboratory in order to understand how Armstrong had been identified amongst the coded samples. The Vrijman (2006) report cleared Armstrong of wrongdoing concluding that his samples had been mishandled, WADA was at fault and that the EPO tests were inadequate for testing purposes. However, it has since been shown that the UCI and Armstrong's legal team were involved in drafting the report aiming to discredit WADA (CIRC, 2015). In 2006, Armstrong was involved in a litigation case with former sponsor SCA Promotions, after the company refused to pay a bonus for winning the 2004

Tour, citing the doping allegations made in *L'Équipe*. Armstrong won the case with a settlement agreed out-of-court, but leaked testimony given by Frankie Andreu, a former teammate, and his wife Betsy Andreu indicated that Armstrong had doped prior to his cancer treatment. This information was again dismissed as there was no evidence to substantiate it.

In May 2010, Floyd Landis, a former teammate of Armstrong and the 2006 Tour de France winner, who was stripped of his title for doping, accused Armstrong of being the head instigator of doping during his time at the US Postal Service Cycling Team and the UCI of covering up Armstrong's doping. At this point, Armstrong had returned to racing and again dismissed the accusations arguing that Landis had no proof. However, Landis' accusations led to the US Justice Department opening an investigation into the claims. The US Justice Department subpoenaed Armstrong's former teammates to give testimony under oath. Additionally, Tyler Hamilton, another of Armstrong's teammates, declared in a CBS interview in 2011 that they had both doped. Hamilton's comments were corroborated by testimonies from other teammates. Despite the testimonies and the evidence collected, the US Justice Department dropped its investigation into Armstrong in February 2012, handing its evidence over to USADA. In June 2012, USADA used the information gained under testimony to formally accuse Armstrong of anti-doping rule violations based on non-analytical data. USADA released a full supporting reasoned decision report in October 2012 that explained its accusations. Armstrong decided not to challenge the accusations, but maintained his innocence, and was consequently stripped of his seven Tour de France titles. He maintained his innocence until January 2013, when, in an interview with US TV show host Oprah Winfrey, Armstrong admitted to doping for much of his career. His ability to evade detection and punishment through a combination of science, subterfuge and bribery created numerous challenges to the propriety of WADA. These questions were propagated long-after his admission of guilt in 2013. For example, the Cycling Independent Reform Commission (CIRC, 2015) report that investigated doping practices in cycling raised further questions about the UCI's relationship with Armstrong.

Such is the significance of Armstrong's case to anti-doping; it has been analysed from multiple academic perspectives. For example, Dimeo (2014) commented that the Armstrong case was unique and represented a confluence of factors including policy change, public interest, federal involvement and USADA ambition. Armstrong's treatment was an exception to previous anti-doping approaches and the zealous, unharmonised approach undermined the legitimacy of the anti-doping system. Armstrong's case has been used to question the legal precedence of USADA and has been related to wider questions of legal proceedings in anti-doping about the burden placed on athletes to prove their innocence (McNamee, 2012). The disparity in treatment again raises questions about the legitimacy of an anti-doping system that is satisfied with settling for a lower standard of guilt than public courts of law which require the prosecutor to demonstrate that the accused is guilty. Other academics have used Armstrong's case to question anti-doping more generally. Sparling (2013) highlighted that 'despite decades of well-intentioned and serious efforts, the current antidoping system is falling short' (p. 3) and required a severe change in approach and attitudes. Likewise, Maennig (2014) used Armstrong's regular deception of testing as an exemplar case of the inefficiency of testing. All these articles shared the same theme that Armstrong's case challenged the legitimacy of the anti-doping system through legal issues and ineffective testing.

Armstrong's case has further been used to exemplify how anti-doping policy approaches could be improved. Bell, Ten Have and Lauchs (2016) proposed that doping involves a network of actors, and WADA's approach to anti-doping should pay closer attention to these key decision-making clusters. They suggested that by targeting key nodes supporting doping networks, such as coaches and suppliers, rather than targeting athletes who are peripheral nodes who can be replaced more easily, anti-doping policy is more likely to have a tangible impact on doping rates. In comparing cases of deliberate professional doping against cases that were accidental, non-performance enhancing, due to medication or at an amateur or master's level, Henning and Dimeo (2014, 2015) used the Armstrong doping case, among other examples, to present how many athletes are becoming 'collateral damage' (2015, p. 405). The authors subsequently recommended that a review of the fairness of anti-doping policy is required and that sanctions need to be developed that have greater sensitivity to the context of doping cases. All of the commentators mentioned here pointed to issues that undermine the legitimacy of WADA, the WADC and the rationale for anti-doping.

Combining academic perspectives on the Armstrong doping case with multilevel legitimacy theory allows two separate issues emerge. The first concerns the continued doping allegations against Armstrong and his ability to avoid detection and punishment. The second concerns information that the UCI had been involved in protecting Armstrong. The following section identifies key periods in Armstrong's case to analyse how it has led to challenges to WADA's legitimacy, and how WADA has responded.

Armstrong, the UCI and WADA: key periods of instability

This section examines the key periods in the two decades that Armstrong's case straddled that challenged WADA's legitimacy and led to the debate. For example, although Floyd Landis' first suggestion that Armstrong had doped in 2010 was a critical turning point in the case, it did not lead to stakeholders challenging WADA specifically. Therefore, we do not consider Landis' action a key period in debates about WADA's legitimacy. Instead, we identify four key periods that generated debate about the legitimacy of WADA: (1) the Vrijman report, (2) Armstrong's decision to stop fighting the doping allegations in 2012,

(3) the first proposed independent commission by the UCI in 2012 and (4) the CIRC report in 2015. The following section discusses each period and analyses the ensuing legitimacy debates.

The first period covers events related to the publication of research in French newspaper *L'Équipe* in 2005 suggesting that Armstrong had used EPO in 1999, and the subsequent investigation led by lawyer Emile Vrijman that cleared Armstrong of any wrongdoing (Vrijman, 2006). The UCI Executive Committee commissioned the investigation to focus specifically on how the information about Armstrong's anti-doping results was leaked from the French anti-doping laboratory to a newspaper and how Armstrong's anonymous samples were identified. Regarding the handling of Armstrong's samples, Vrijman concluded: 'Sometimes with doping cases you can say it was a technicality. These are not technicalities. These are fundamental issues which should have been done differently' (Vrijman, 2006). WADA wanted the investigation to include whether Armstrong had committed any wrongdoing (i.e., doped). Ultimately, UCI executives used the report to challenge the performance of WADA as the anti-doping system had leaked the private information. WADA responded by attacking the credibility of the report. This escalated when the incumbent WADA President, Dick Pound, engaged in a verbal argument with Armstrong.

The second period relevant to WADA's legitimacy was Armstrong's decision to stop fighting the doping allegations put forward by USADA in 2012. This period followed the decision by the U.S. Department of Justice to stop investigating claims put forward by Floyd Landis about doping during Armstrong's time on a professional cycling team sponsored by the U.S. Postal Service. Importantly, during this investigation, 12 witness testimonies were gained under oath from Armstrong's teammates and assistants, which were later passed onto USADA. USADA used these testimonies to prosecute Armstrong, releasing the details of the decision in a reasoned report (USADA, 2012). Following USADA's decision to prosecute Armstrong, WADA was challenged by UCI representatives for conducting a witch-hunt on Armstrong, and cycling in general. The UCI's protest was met with a defiant response from WADA executives who denied the claims. When USADA's reasoned decision was published, it provided evidence that Armstrong and the UCI had undermined and evaded WADA's testing regime, posing significant concerns about the anti-doping system to which the organisation was forced to respond.

The third event that led to debate over the legitimacy of WADA was the first Independent Commission proposed by then UCI President Patrick McQuaid in late 2012. The Commission was designed to investigate the actions of Armstrong. However, the remit of the Commission was criticised by WADA for not investigating the alleged complicity of the UCI staff in helping Armstrong avoid detection. This again led to conflict between the UCI Executive Committee which had challenged WADA's lack of support for the commission and WADA which publicly attacked the UCI's integrity.

The fourth event was the publication of the CIRC report (2015). The CIRC report was commissioned by the new UCI President, Brian Cookson, in 2013. Cookson's election as UCI President began a new period of reconciliation between WADA and the UCI, as the report was given scope to investigate the actions of the former UCI Presidents Hein Verbruggen (1991–2005) and Patrick McQuaid (2005–2013). The report challenged WADA's legitimacy, highlighting deficiencies in its testing quality as well as its inability to control sociocultural factors, such as the mafia-style 'Omerta' (i.e., the collective tendency for cyclists to remain silent about doping and outcast those who do speak up). WADA responded with manipulation, claiming that the report's findings constituted an achievement much like the USADA's reasoned decision. Three key discussion points emerge from this case pertinent to how WADA's legitimacy was contested: (1) the victimisation of Armstrong and the UCI, (2) WADA attacking the source of challenges and (3) reinterpreting exposed testing inefficiencies to gain further regulatory powers.

Victimisation

Throughout the case UCI executives and Armstrong portrayed themselves as being unfairly treated and victimised by WADA, which they used as a platform to challenge WADA's legitimacy. Adopting the position of the victim allowed the UCI executives and Armstrong to voice negative judgements of WADA. The imposition of anti-doping policy created by WADA in the first WADC in 2003 did not appear to provide any benefit to Armstrong or the UCI Executive Committee. Improved testing standards stipulated in the WADC posed a risk to the success of Armstrong, and by proxy, the commercial ambitions of the UCI, if testing demonstrated that doping was widespread. The threat of anti-doping to the UCI and Armstrong was expressed in negative legitimacy judgements towards WADA.

There are multiple examples from the four periods previously identified where UCI executives and Armstrong voiced negative judgements about WADA. Following accusations in L'Équipe that one of Armstrong's blood samples had tested positive for EPO, both Armstrong and the UCI challenged the credibility of the French Laboratory accredited by WADA. For example, Armstrong questioned the ethics of the French Anti-Doping laboratory arguing that 'there's a setup here and I'm stuck in the middle of it. I absolutely do not trust that laboratory' (Vertuno, 2005). In a separate interview he reiterated his scepticism:

> Protocol was not followed and there's no back up sample to confirm what they say. So why are six of them positive and the other 11 aren't? I'm saying there were 17 samples. So, if the drug would stay around for two, three, four weeks, we have 17 samples given, and only six of them positive. What happened to the other 11?

> ('Anti-doping body', 2005, August 26)

Armstrong questioned how the allegations could be correct if testing had never previously identified him. Either the previous testing was inadequate, or the results were incorrect. Furthermore, he linked this point to a lack of trust in the testers if they had leaked information to the press. Of course, it was in Armstrong's self-interest to discredit the legitimacy of WADA's new testing. The UCI executives would have also benefited from a negative consensus about the legitimacy of WADA's testing regime as it may have given them the opportunity to take back control of drug testing in cycling. This was demonstrated by a UCI press release that was critical of WADA:

> We have substantial concerns about the impact of this matter on the integrity of the overall drug testing regime of the Olympic movement, and in particular the questions it raises over the trustworthiness of some of the sports and political authorities active in the anti-doping fight.
>
> (Harnischfger, 2005, September 9)

Following the publication of the Vrijman report clearing Armstrong of wrongdoing, he maintained his challenge to the performance of WADA's testing regime: 'The report confirms my innocence but also finds that Mr. Pound [WADA President, Dick Pound] along with the French lab and the French ministry have ignored the rules and broken the law' (Halliburton, 2006, June 1). Armstrong went further challenging WADA's performance in controlling the laboratories it accredits:

> It's shocking to me that Mr. Pound, and the people at WADA, the lab, the ministry, the organizers view the system as a unilateral system. The word control doesn't just apply to the athletes. The word control has to apply to the police, too, and to the organizers and the media.
>
> (Litke, 2006, June 2)

The UCI Executive Committee reiterated a failing in performance declaring: 'The UCI reminds that this report exposes the irregularities committed by WADA and does not bring any other proof that Lance Armstrong had violated the anti-doping rules and regulations' (Jones, 2006, June 2). The theme throughout these challenges was that Armstrong had been unfairly treated by the anti-doping system, as rules had been broken which enabled both parties to then challenge WADA.

The suggestion of unfair treatment was characteristic of the UCI Executive Committee and Armstrong during other time periods as well. After Armstrong was charged by USADA with an ADRV, rather than giving evidence to discredit the allegations, he doubted the anti-doping prosecution system. His argument relied on the assertion that he would not be treated fairly:

> If I thought for one moment that by participating in USADA's process I could confront these allegations in a fair setting and, once and for all, put

these charges to rest, I would jump at the chance. I refuse to participate in a process that is so one-sided and unfair.

(Carter, 2012, August 23)

Similarly, following USADA's decision to charge Armstrong, UCI President Patrick McQuaid challenged prejudices in WADA's Executive Committee: 'Historically over the past 10 or 15 years there has been a political campaign against cycling by senior people within WADA and I don't think that's acceptable' (Sweeney, 2012, August 26). Even after Armstrong's confession, the UCI management maintained that they had been unfairly singled out when defending their first Independent Commission (that was later disbanded). They challenged WADA's testing arguing, 'USADA and WADA also tested Armstrong over many years and also failed to catch him. It was only with the benefit of the US federal investigation that USADA was finally able to gain evidence of Armstrong's doping' (Munnery, 2013, April 26). Both the UCI Executive Committee and Armstrong used the events to portray themselves as being subject to unfair treatment and to undermine WADA's legitimacy.

Evidence in CIRC (2015) suggested that during the years that the UCI protected Armstrong, the priority social values held by the UCI Executive Committee focused on promoting the sport through the celebrity appeal of Armstrong, even if this meant ignoring ADRVs. For example, the report stated: 'The emphasis of UCI's anti-doping policy was to give the impression that UCI was tough on doping rather than actually being good at anti-doping' (CIRC, 2015, p. 10). A source in the CIRC claimed: 'The primary concern was the commercial and international development of cycling, and the arrival of Lance Armstrong was an extraordinary opportunity, a real success story, and the UCI closed its eyes to the rest' (p. 197). Therefore, WADA's legitimacy would be judged in relation to such commercial imperatives. The UCI Executive Committee and Armstrong used their position as a victim to voice challenges that questioned WADA's purpose.

In 2003, UCI President Hein Verbruggen (1991–2005) claimed that WADA and its President Dick Pound exceeded its regulatory authority and accused Pound of 'behaving like a Sheriff in the Wild West' (Kernaghan, 2003). After the publication of the Vrijman report, Armstrong wrote to former IOC President, Jacques Rogge to complain about Pound: 'Ever since WADA was created, Dick Pound has been criticized for improperly using his position to attack athletes and sports organisations without evidence and for making statements about athletes' guilt without any evidence to support his statements' (Zinser, 2006, August 8). All these challenges insinuated that WADA had extended its actions beyond its remit of regulation and was interfering in sport. By doing so it conflicted with the UCI's apathetic anti-doping efforts at the time.

Criticisms were also evident after WADA's refusal to support the Independent Commission proposed by the UCI in 2013. The UCI President McQuaid argued that WADA unfairly targeted the UCI:

The UCI is perplexed that WADA has now chosen to rebuff and attack the UCI's willingness to establish a truth and reconciliation commission, having just demanded that the UCI establish exactly such a commission. I would therefore urge the President of WADA one more time to try to set his personal vendetta and crusade against cycling aside and to support the UCI in doing what is right for cycling.

(Mark, 2013, January 30)

McQuaid's statement implied that the UCI was being victimised by WADA to the detriment of anti-doping efforts in cycling. After the commission was abandoned, McQuaid went on to place the blame on WADA:

I am sorry that it has to be abandoned but we could not afford the money that we wanted to spend on it and, having the report for just one side and the fact neither WADA nor USADA were prepared to collaborate to this commission, put us in a situation where we had no option but to cancel it and look at a different approach.

('Nothing to hide', 2013, May 24)

The statement implied that it was WADA's fault for the lack of an investigation designed to improve anti-doping. The use of victimisation as a position for institutional change is novel. Typically, research has focused on field position, power and resource differences to explain sources of institutional change. However, the evidence presented in the next section suggests that portraying oneself as a victim is not a strong position from which to challenge the legitimacy of institutions given that WADA was able to defy the challenges. Furthermore, it appeared that stakeholders could adopt a public moral stance that may be incongruent with internal organisational beliefs to challenge an institution's legitimacy. For instance, it was evident that the UCI Executive Committee and Armstrong did not morally value anti-doping, but by pretending to be troubled by WADA's lack of support for their supposed stance on anti-doping, they were able to challenge the organisation.

Attacking the source

It was apparent that throughout the Armstrong case, WADA staff adopted a defiant stance in response to the challenges launched by the UCI Executive Committee and Armstrong. In particular, WADA staff attacked the credibility of their challengers. Oliver (1991) argued that attacking defiance is a 'strive to assault, belittle, or vehemently denounce institutionalized values and the external constituents that express them' (p. 157). In effect, there was a relationship between the legitimacy of WADA and the challenger. When actors criticised WADA, the organisation subsequently sought to undermine the perceived credibility of the challenger.

The challenges levelled at WADA were highly critical. When the UCI Executive Committee and Armstrong challenged WADA following the *L'Équipe* article, Pound voiced his complaints against the UCI investigation in a WADA Executive Committee meeting in November (WADA, 2005):

> [WADA] did not know how the particular lawyer had been chosen for this; it did not know as much as it would like to about the lawyer selected; it did not know the terms of reference; and it could not get any answers to its correspondence on this, so WADA did not know whether or not it was a real investigation, and it did not know whether there was any interest in a full investigation.
>
> (WADA, 2005)

In addition, statements in the Vrijman report (2006) accused WADA of wrongdoing. For example, Vrijman claimed: 'The refusal by the Laboratoire National de Détection du Dopage (LNDD), the French Ministry and WADA to provide documents and information that are necessary for the proper conduct of a complete investigation is extremely troubling and is inconsistent with the principles of the Olympic Movement' (Vrijman, 2006, p. 16). As previously noted, the UCI Executive Committee and Armstrong used the report to challenge WADA's legitimacy. WADA's response vigorously attacked the claims as they 'completely rejected the report' ("Armstrong report rejected", 2006). Pound declared that the report 'bordered on the farcical' (Gillon, 2006, June 24) and had a 'distinct lack of impartiality in conducting a full review of all the facts' (Myles, 2006, June 28). Pound later attacked the UCI's legitimacy to comment on doping declaring that 'there is no sport that is immune but cycling certainly has a high proportion of doping' (Fotheringham, 2006, July 28).

The poor relationship between the UCI Executive Committee, Armstrong and WADA was evident throughout the period following USADA's decision to charge Armstrong. Following Armstrong's refusal to engage in the anti-doping process to defend his innocence, WADA president John Fahey initially defended the system: 'I am confident and WADA is confident that the USADA acted within the WADA code, and that a court in Texas also decided not to interfere' (Zennie, 2012, August 24). Fahey also attacked Armstrong's decision: 'He had a right to contest the charges. He chose not to. The simple fact is that his refusal to examine the evidence means the charges had substance in them' ('USADA strips Armstrong', 2012, August 24). When UCI resident McQuaid highlighted Armstrong's unfair treatment by suggesting he had 'a trial in the court of public opinion' (Sweeney, 2012, August 26), David Howman, Director General of WADA, attacked the UCI Executive Committee: 'By adopting its current position, UCI is sadly destroying the credibility it has been slowly regaining in the past years in the fight against doping' (Sweeney, 2012, August 26).

Following the UCI Executive Committee's first attempt to establish an Independent Commission to investigate doping, WADA refused to lend support as it believed it needed a broader scope to look at doping in cycling more generally. Fahey commented: 'Instead UCI has again chosen to ignore its responsibility to the sport of cycling in completing such an inquiry and has determined to apparently deflect responsibility for the doping problem in its sport to others' (WADA, 2013b). He further questioned the federation's commitment to anti-doping. Given that the UCI President McQuaid challenged the legitimacy of WADA by placing the responsibility for the commission's eventual failure on WADA (Mark, 2013, January 30), John Fahey countered by laying the blame on the UCI President for making the inquiry's focus to narrow and refusing to extend the scope: 'WADA has been informed that the commission and UCI are not willing to change the terms of reference and timetable, and for this reason WADA has declined to spend money and dedicate resources on an inquiry that has such obvious limitations' (WADA, 2013a). Fahey's statement reiterated that the UCI was at fault and that no credence should be given to the previous Vrijman report discrediting the UCI and Armstrong's challenges:

> It has again become apparent that rather than deal with the obvious problems that exist within the sport of cycling, the UCI once again would like to avoid its responsibilities and instead seek to blame WADA and others. This is not the first time that the UCI has acted in this way. In 2005 when an opportunity arose to address an allegation of doping by Armstrong, the UCI commissioned a so-called independent report – the Vrijman Report – which totally failed to address the substance of the allegations against Armstrong.
>
> (WADA, 2013a)

When the Commission was finally axed, a UCI press statement reasoned that WADA's lack of assistance was the reason for it being disbanded. Again, Fahey countered the UCI Executive Committee and suggested they were lying:

> WADA has not and will not consider partaking in any venture with UCI while this unilateral and arrogant attitude continues. There has been no suggestion made by WADA that it will pay for or contribute to any collaborative effort with UCI into investigating UCI's long-standing problems with doping in its sport and its alleged complicity.
>
> (Gibson, 2013, January 29)

Armstrong was not immune to criticism from WADA representatives in the period following his interview with Oprah Winfrey in which he claimed to have doped to level the playing field. Armstrong's claim that doping was widespread insinuated that WADA had failed to control doping in cycling, an assertion that was refuted by WADA staff. For example, Fahey claimed that it was 'a convenient way of justifying what he did' ('Armstrong admits doping', 2013, January 18), and David Howman added: 'It seemed to us it was more of a convenient truth than a full display of what went on and that is really what we would ask him to do' ('Ducking, diving and deceit', 2013, January 19).

Our discussion of how WADA attacked the challenger illustrates how the organisation attempted to discredit the source of legitimacy challenges. When faced with legitimacy challenges demanding behavioural change that may require substantial work, or that are incompatible with the aims of the organisation, discrediting the source of the legitimacy challenge via attacking defiance may provide a more viable option. A savvier organisation challenging the legitimacy of WADA may have pointed out that the organisation's defiance failed to address the challenges raised about testing and integrity, and that the source of the challenge should be irrelevant if the issue raised is genuine (i.e., performance challenges to testing). McNamee (2012) argued that Armstrong's case, irrelevant of guilt, was not passable in a court of law by accepted practices of law, so why should anti-doping maintain different standards. We suggest that the reluctance of other stakeholders to publicly support the UCI and Armstrong in challenging WADA may indicate the presence of suppressor factors that made it risky to disagree with the consensus of validity around WADA's legitimacy. By supporting the UCI (an organisation with a poor record on anti-doping), organisations may have found themselves suffering reputational damage through association.

Reinterpreting testing inefficiencies

The final issue in this chapter concerns how WADA has, in addition to attacking the source of challenges, strived to manipulate and influence the expectations of stakeholders. The Armstrong case provided evidence that drug testing could be beaten via science and human corruption. Previous research has used Armstrong's case to illustrate that testing has been ineffective at delivering doping-free sport (Maennig, 2014; Sparling, 2013). As Armstrong himself pointed out, 'I was caught, but 99 other times, I wasn't. Riders think they can get away with doping because most of the time they do' (Moore, 2012). Armstrong was eventually charged with ADRVs based on witness testimonies given under oath obtained from a US Federal investigation (USADA, 2012). WADA's inability to catch Armstrong through testing alone highlighted the deficiencies in the system. Yet, WADA reinterpreted this reality to promote the need for greater cooperation with investigative authorities (e.g., Interpol) and to justify new powers in the WADC to launch its own investigations. From this perspective, WADA actively shifted what evaluators might judge as legitimate behaviour, moving from an organisation originally created with a regulatory and monitoring capacity to an organisation with investigatory powers.

Following the first edition of the WADC, WADA's focus on testing came under challenge at the time of the L'Équipe article and the Vrijman Report. For example, former WADA Athlete Committee member Becky Scott explained: 'There are still a lot of holes in the testing and policing system that need to be sealed up before we can say an athlete is clean even if they have passed their tests' (Morris, 2005, August 24). Armstrong commented that 'the actual test for EPO, what they call electrophoresis, is actually being questioned on a pretty serious level right now. Why do you think they're still working on it? Because it doesn't work that well' (King, 2005, August 25). Later, the Vrijman report concluded that it was 'completely irresponsible for anyone involved in doping control to even suggest that the analyses results that were reported constitute evidence of anything' (Vrijman, 2006, p. 17). Even though the Vrijman report was compromised by interference (CIRC, 2015), this period presented a series of challenges to WADA's early strategic focus on testing.

WADA's change in tactics was evident from the discourse it promoted prior to and following the USADA report. In discussing the role of federal authorities in the doping case of Armstrong as well as US sprinter Marion Jones, WADA Director General David Howman alluded to the benefits of greater cooperation:

> What we do now is we don't just rely on testing. We don't just rely on getting samples and sending them to the lab. We rely a lot more, in addition, on these inquiries where the police in all the countries can get information that we can't get through the science.
>
> (Marantz, 2011, June 1)

When the US Federal investigation into Armstrong was terminated, John Fahey stated in reference to the information obtained under oath that it would be 'very, very helpful if that information was handed over' ('WADA seeks new probe', 2012, February 9). Following the publication of the USADA (2012) report, the following statement from Howman was indicative of how WADA turned testing failures into a win for investigation powers:

> Do I think that a conspiracy of this sort could prevail now? No I don't. This started in pre-WADA days because the WADA Code did not come into effect until 2004. There has been a change of approach that has come about in the last four or five years in relation to not only gathering evidence through sample analysis but also through other means. This case is a good example of those other means showing that cheats can't avoid detection simply by manipulating the sample process. Five years ago we linked up with Interpol and now we've linked up with customs. If you're going to be strong on getting rid of cheats in sport, you've got to use all the available resources.
>
> (Hart, 2012, October 12)

It appears that the effectiveness of intelligence and investigations in catching Armstrong was able to support a growing case from WADA to have an investigatory capacity. John Fahey echoed Howman's comments on the value of intelligence and investigations:

This was simply a painstaking investigation by an anti-doping body. Not by a law-enforcement body. And full credit for the detail they went into, and the manner in which they corroborated evidence from witness after witness, to piece together a damning account which has shocked the world.

(Payten, 2012, October 20)

The strongest evidence that WADA leveraged the Armstrong case to gain investigatory powers comes from the comments of Fahey about the proposed changes to the 2015 WADC:

The proposal that goes out in December clearly articulates that WADA has the power to investigate. What that tells me is that when a sporting body, an anti-doping organization is given information and they do nothing about it - and we've had many examples of that in the past - that WADA can go in and do something about it with investigative powers.

('WADA proposes', 2012, November 19)

Favourably for WADA, the Armstrong case also coincided with the WADC progress review. Reflecting upon Armstrong, the BALCO scandal and Operation Puerto (a doping investigation into Spanish doctor Eufemiano Fuentes), all anti-doping investigations that had uncovered athletes who were not being detected by tests, Fahey asserted: 'Investigations, in particular, are seen as essential if we are to do what we must do as effectively as we can' ('Four-year bans', 2013, November 15).

The impact of the investigations approach championed after the case of Armstrong had a significant impact on the CIRC report as well. For example, at both the formation and publication of CIRC, WADA gave its support for this investigative approach. When CIRC was formed, WADA expressed its faith in investigations (WADA, 2014). In addition, when the CIRC report was published, WADA reiterated its support for the UCI's investigative approach into retrospective issues: 'The Commission should be commended for their extensive investigation into the historical problems relating to the sport of cycling and for the thoroughness of their Report' (WADA, 2015).

WADA's ability to influence institutional processes to increase its capacities should not be underestimated. During the Essendon Football Club investigation (this is discussed in greater detail in chapter seven) in the AFL, Fahey used the Armstrong case to justify the time and resources being spent on the investigation: 'The findings will come when they come. It took two years in America to get to the point where charges were laid against Lance Armstrong and others' (Lane, 2013, August 1). It was noted by Fahey that the lawyer Richard Young, who aided USADA in catching Armstrong, was also involved in the Essendon investigation, and that his 'expertise was critical to Australian Sport Anti-doping Agency's work regarding the investigation' (Lane, 2014, June 15). This strategy appeared to be a deliberate attempt by WADA to support its attempts to change the expected legitimate behaviour of WADA to include facilitating investigations.

The effectiveness of WADA's manipulation tactics were evident in other recent high-profile doping cases. Concerns about the quality of testing have not disappeared as demonstrated by the disparity in athletes sanctioned and athletes who admit to using PEDs (e.g., Ulrich et al., 2018). That the Russian Olympic doping scandal (discussed in greater detail in chapter nine) was also exposed due to whistle-blowers and followed up by large-scale investigations signified that testing remains vulnerable to subterfuge. In addition to concerns about testing, the UCI's actions demonstrated the conflicts of interest placed upon international federations implementing testing. The WADC testing regime is dependent upon signatories who find themselves conflicted between policing sport and promoting sport. Under the WADC, testing will only ever be as effective as the efforts of the signatories that are responsible for managing anti-doping. The recent introduction of the International Testing Agency (ITA) to manage anti-doping testing processes for events and international federations may offer a solution to the kind of corruption seen in the Armstrong case by separating responsibility for testing from signatories.

Conclusion

In conclusion, our analysis of the Lance Armstrong case focused on three key insights into the legitimacy of WADA. The first point, 'victimisation' drew together arguments that the UCI Executive Committee members and Armstrong framed their challenges by positioning themselves as victims of unfair treatment by WADA. In doing so they justified their judgements, which may have been based upon perceptions that promoting cycling should be prioritised over anti-doping efforts. The second point, 'attacking the source', demonstrated that WADA has predominantly responded to legitimacy challenges by attacking the UCI and Armstrong's credibility. This response style sought to discredit the source rather than answer the criteria of the challenge. Given cycling's previous poor record on regulating anti-doping, WADA may have recognised this was a better option than trying to meet the demands of the challenge or at least avoid or manipulate them. The third point, 'reinterpreting testing inefficiencies' argued that WADA used the case of Armstrong to strengthen its own capabilities despite being shown to be inefficient at delivering clean sport through testing. Using Armstrong's case as leverage, as well as other successful investigations into doping such as the BALCO scandal and Operation Puerto, WADA was able to authorise investigatory capabilities in the 2015 edition of the WADC, which consequently gave them the ability to launch investigations. The omission from this argument, however, is that these investigations caught athletes after they were successful. Catching an athlete who has doped a long time after he or she has won and deprived other competitor following the rules may be of little value to the opponent who is retrospectively awarded the victory.

In relation to our broader aim, this case contributes to a growing narrative about WADA. Firstly, Armstrong's case suggests that when the legitimacy of WADA is challenged, it can use the event to increase its organisational capabilities via reinterpreting shortcomings as opportunities for development. In the same way that WADA has progressively expected more whereabouts information from athletes, this change to investigations evidences how WADA has increased its control over anti-doping and how an institution can reinforce itself after a period of instability. Secondly, the legitimacy of the source that creates a challenge appears to be significant for garnering further support. In challenges related to the whereabouts system, federations were able to take cues from each other to question issues at a higher level. However, in this instance, the UCI was isolated in questioning the behaviour of WADA and the efficacy of testing. Finally, building on the findings of the whereabouts case study, defiance and manipulation were common responses from WADA to legitimacy challenges, suggesting a pattern of resistance to challenge rather than acquiescence. Chapter six will continue our exploration of the legitimacy of WADA by analysing the therapeutic use exemption system. By exploring the relationship between the therapeutic use exemption system and WADA's legitimacy, we provide further insight into WADA's defiant approach.

References

Anti-doping body sent Lance tests. (2005, August 26). Retrieved from https://edition. cnn.com/.

Armstrong admits doping: 'I'm a flawed character'. (2013, January 18). *The Bangkok Post*. Retrieved from https://www.bangkokpost.com/.

Armstrong report rejected. (2006, June 3). *Pittsburgh Post Gazette*. Retrieved from http:// www.post-gazette.com/.

Bell, P., Ten Have, C., & Lauchs, M. (2016). A case study analysis of a sophisticated sports doping network: Lance Armstrong and the USPS Team. *International Journal of Law, Crime and Justice, 46*, 57–68.

Carter, C. (2012, August 23). Lance Armstrong facing lifetime ban. *CNN*. Retrieved from https://edition.cnn.com/.

CIRC. (2015). Report to the president of the Union Cycliste Internationale. *Cycling Independent Reform Commission*. Switzerland: Lausanne.

Dimeo, P. (2014). Why Lance Armstrong? Historical context and key turning points in the 'cleaning up' of professional cycling. *The International Journal of the History of Sport, 31*(8), 951–968.

Ducking, diving and deceit prove to be difficult habits for serial cheat to break. (2013, January 19). *The Irish Times*. Retrieved from https://www.irishtimes.com/.

Fotheringham, S. (2006, July 28). Tour title put on hold as Landis fails drugs test. *The Guardian*. Retrieved from https://www.theguardian.com/uk.

Four-year bans for doping cheats passed by global sports watchdog. (2013, November 15). *The Record*. Retrieved from https://www.therecord.com/.

Gibson, O. (2013, January 29). WADA 'dismayed' by UCI's handling of Lance Armstrong fallout. *The Guardian*. Retrieved from https://www.theguardian.com/uk.

Gillon, D. (2006, June 24). Tour legend Armstrong faces fresh drug allegations. *The Scotland Herald.* Retrieved from https://www.heraldscotland.com/.

Halliburton, S. (2006, June 1). Again, he emerges victorious. *The New Statesman.* Retrieved from https://www.statesman.com/.

Hambrick, M.E., Frederick, E.L., & Sanderson, J. (2015). From yellow to blue: Exploring Lance Armstrong's image repair strategies across traditional and social media. *Communication & Sport, 3*(2), 196–218.

Harnischfger, U. (2005, September 9). Cycling body criticizes world doping authorities, French newspaper over Armstrong allegations. *The Associated Press.* Retrieved from https://www.ap.org/en-us/.

Hart, S. (2012, October 12). Drug conspiracy 'not possible' in present climate. *The Telegraph.* Retrieved from https://www.telegraph.co.uk/.

Henning, A.D. & Dimeo, P. (2014). The complexities of anti-doping violations: A case study of sanctioned cases in all performance levels of USA cycling. *Performance Enhancement & Health, 3*(3–4), 159–166.

Henning, A.D., & Dimeo, P. (2015). Questions of fairness and anti-doping in US cycling: The contrasting experiences of professionals and amateurs. *Drugs: Education, Prevention and Policy, 22*(5), 400–409.

Jones, J. (2006, June 2). UCI supports Vrijman's findings. *Cycling News.* Retrieved from http://autobus.cyclingnews.com/.

Kernaghan, J. (2003). Cycling tires of getting pounded. *The Spectator.* Retrieved from https://www.thespec.com/.

King, L. (2005, August 25). *Interview with Lance Armstrong.* Retrieved from https://edition.cnn.com/.

Lane, S. (2013, August 1). Drug probe has no time limit: Fahey. *Sunday Morning Herald.* Retrieved from https://www.smh.com.au/.

Lane, S. (2014, June 15). Dons drug case invokes Armstrong. *Sydney Morning Herald.* Retrieved from https://www.smh.com.au/.

Litke, J. (2006, June 2). Armstrong keeps suspicion in rearview mirror. *The Monterey Herald.* Retrieved from https://www.montereyherald.com/.

Maennig, W. (2014). Inefficiency of the anti-doping system: Cost reduction proposals. *Substance Use & Misuse, 49*(9), 1201–1205.

Marantz, K. (2011, June 1). Lance and the art of denial. *The Japan News.* Retrieved from http://the-japan-news.com/.

Mark, D. (2013, January 30). UCI and WADA spat over abandoned drug commission. *ABC.* Retrieved from http://www.abc.net.au/.

McNamee, M. (2012). Lance Armstrong, anti-doping policy, and the need for ethical commentary by philosophers of sport. *Sports, Ethics and Philosophy, 6*(3), 305–307.

Moore, O. (2012, October 19). Seven ways to cheat the tests. *The Globe and Mail.* Retrieved from https://www.theglobeandmail.com/.

Morris, J. (2005, August 24). Onus now on Lance to prove he's clean. *The Edmonton Journal.* Retrieved from https://edmontonjournal.com/.

Munnery, S. (2013, April 26). UCI hits back at Travis Tygart over allegations of Armstrong cover-up. *The Times.* Retrieved from https://www.thetimes.co.uk.

Myles, S. (2006, June 28). Progress made in ferreting out cheats. *The Montreal Gazette.* Retrieved from https://montrealgazette.com/.

Nothing to hide over Armstrong. (2013, May 24). *Bangkok Post*. Retrieved from https://www.bangkokpost.com/.

Oliver, C. (1991). Strategic responses to institutional processes. *Academy of Management Review, 16*(1), 145–179.

Payten, I. (2012, October 20). Landing the biggest fish doesn't mean there aren't a lot more out there. *The Telegraph*. Retrieved from https://www.dailytelegraph.com.au/.

Sparling, P.B. (2013). The Lance Armstrong saga: A wake-up call for drug reform in sports. *Current Sports Medicine Reports, 12*(2), 53–54.

Sweeney, E. (2012, August 26). Truth wins out in the end. *The Irish Independent*. Retrieved from https://www.independent.ie/.

Ulrich, R., Pope, H.G., Cléret, L., Petróczi, A., Nepusz, T., Schaffer, J., ... & Simon, P. (2018). Doping in two elite athletics competitions assessed by randomized-response surveys. *Sports Medicine, 48*(1), 211–219.

USADA. (2012). Report on Proceedings under the World Anti-Doping Code and the USADA Protocol; United States Anti-Doping Agency, Claimant v. Lance Armstrong, Respondent; Reasoned Decision of the United States Anti-Doping Agency on Disqualification and Ineligibility. Retrieved from http://cyclinginvestigation.usada.org/.

USADA strips Armstrong of Tour de France titles. (2012, August 24). *RTE*. Retrieved from https://www.rte.ie/news/.

Vertuno, J. (2005, August 25). Armstrong says he's victim of 'setup'. *The Associated Press*. Retrieved from https://www.ap.org/en-us/.

Vrijman, E. (2006). Independent investigation analysis samples from the 1999 Tour de France. Retrieved from http://velorooms.com/files/Vrijman-Report-full.pdf.

WADA. (2005, November 20). Executive Committee meeting minutes. Retrieved from https://www.wada-ama.org/en.

WADA. (2013a). WADA will not partake in UCI Independent Commission. Retrieved from https://www.wada-ama.org/en.

WADA. (2013b). Statement from WADA President John Fahey in response to UCI press release of January 28, 2013. World Anti-Doping Agency. Retrieved from https://www.wada-ama.org/.

WADA. (2014). WADA statement on Cycling Independent Reform Commission. Retrieved from https://www.wada-ama.org/en.

WADA. (2015). WADA Director General Statement on the Cycling Independent Reform Commission report. Retrieved from https://www.wada-ama.org/en.

WADA proposes tougher doping sanctions. (2012, November 19). *Bangkok Post*. Retrieved from https://www.bangkokpost.com/.

WADA seeks new probe of Armstrong evidence. (2012, February 9). *The Mercury*. Retrieved from https://www.themercury.com.au/.

Zennie, M. (2012, August 24). Banned for life! Disgraced Lance Armstrong STRIPPED of seven Tour de France titles as he stops fighting doping charges. *The Daily Mail*. Retrieved from https://www.dailymail.co.uk/home/index.html.

Zinser, L. (2006, August 8). Pound builds and badgers in his battle against doping. *The New York Times*. Retrieved from https://www.nytimes.com/.

Chapter 6

Therapeutic use exemptions

The ability for athletes to take medical substances that are otherwise prohibited has, for some stakeholders, been a contentious issue for the legitimacy of anti-doping policy under World Anti-Doping Agency (WADA). Therapeutic use exemptions (TUEs) are a cornerstone of anti-doping policy that permit professional athletes medical treatment with otherwise prohibited substances. The WADC (2020) states that:

> The presence of a Prohibited Substance or its Metabolites or Markers, and/ or the Use or Attempted Use, Possession or Administration or Attempted Administration of a Prohibited Substance or Prohibited Method shall not be considered an anti-doping rule violation if it is consistent with the provisions of a TUE granted in accordance with the International Standard for Therapeutic Use Exemptions. (p. 35)

To this point we have demonstrated that WADA's legitimacy is tied to how stakeholders evaluate the organisation's policies and subsequent responses, as we demonstrated in chapter four when analysing the whereabouts system. The TUE system has created similar problems as the rule has created legitimacy challenges for WADA. The TUE rule reinterprets the line of acceptable drug use to include potentially performance-enhancing substances if athletes have a medical need, thereby affording opportunities for misuse. For example, elite athletes in sports with a high aerobic demand are at greater risk of developing asthma (Selge, Thomas, Nowak, Radon, & Wolfarth, 2016), therefore, is the use of prohibited corticosteroids to treat their condition unfair, even if they do not offer performance-enhancing benefits when taken at therapeutic levels? Likewise, is a marathon runner using an analgesic substance to mask pain and compete whilst injured 'unnaturally' enhancing his or her performance above what it would be without medication, or is he or she just returning to a pre-injury state? Answering these questions depends largely upon a policy interpretation about what constitutes doping. Since WADA formulates and implements a unilateral policy interpretation concerning what doping entails, the administration and misuse of the TUE rule reflect directly upon its legitimacy.

The TUE rule was first introduced by the IOC in 1992, but its incorporation into the WADC by WADA facilitated global recognition and adoption (Fitch, 2013). WADA laid out standards to ensure that the TUE process was consistent and fair across sports and nations including (1) the need for NADOs to create a TUE committee responsible for granting exemptions with at least three experts in clinical, sports and exercise medicine of whom at least two are independent; (2) the need for NADOs to report all TUE decisions to WADA; and (3) the ability for WADA to review TUE committee decisions in certain circumstances (WADA, 2020). Example of TUEs include the permitted use of corticosteroid-based medication for asthma treatment or sympathomimetic psychostimulants (e.g., Ritalin) for attention deficit hyperactivity disorder. Importantly, applications for the use of certain prohibited substances with a proven performance-enhancing effect (e.g., β-blockers) can still be rejected even if the medical condition is valid (Pike, 2018).

To analyse how the TUE system has generated legitimacy challenges, this chapter is structured as follows. Firstly, previous discussions of the TUE system are presented with a specific focus on the TUE process in order to provide an explanation of the rules underpinning the system. Secondly, five critical periods related to the TUE system which have led to WADA's legitimacy being challenged are outlined, including both athlete and organisational examples. Lastly, three points are examined in relation to WADA's legitimacy: (1) *accuracy of diagnosis* pertaining to practical challenges with TUE implementation, (2) *moral ambiguity* which refers to arguments about the appropriateness of TUE in sport and (3) the *political opportunism* visible around the TUE rule.

Therapeutic use exemptions: legal doping?

The incoming 2021 International Standard for TUE (WADA, 2020, p. 10–11) states that a TUE may be granted if, on the balance of probabilities, the following criteria are satisfied:

A. The Prohibited Substance or Prohibited Method in question is needed to treat a diagnosed medical condition supported by relevant clinical evidence.
B. The Therapeutic Use of the Prohibited Substance or Prohibited Method will not, on the balance of probabilities, produce any additional enhancement of performance beyond what might be anticipated by a return to the Athlete's normal state of health following the treatment of the medical condition.
C. The Prohibited Substance or Prohibited Method is an indicated treatment for the medical condition, and there is no reasonable permitted Therapeutic alternative.
D. The necessity for the Use of the Prohibited Substance or Prohibited Method is not a consequence, wholly or in part, of the prior Use (without a TUE) of a substance or method which was prohibited at the time of such Use.

If these criteria are not satisfactorily fulfilled or the TUE committee rules that the substance is not appropriate, a TUE will not be granted. In theory, by meeting the criteria listed here, the potential for misuse is limited as TUEs will only be given to those athletes who need them for legitimate medical purposes. However, differences in prescribing and treatment trends, and medication availability globally, can create problematic inconsistencies.

The TUE rule has been subject to debate primarily due to concerns about the robustness of the TUE process (e.g., Lentillon-Kaestner, Hagger, & Hardcastle, 2012; Pitsiladis et al., 2017). For instance, the process could be undermined by medical professionals who incorrectly diagnose athletes with certain conditions, so that healthy athletes have access to medications with performance-enhancing effects. This would violate criteria A of the International Standard for TUE. Equally, each physician could employ a different prescription policy, while athletes could practice variable treatment habits. In addition, harmonised TUE application decision-making globally presents further challenges to the system (Hughes et al., 2020). As a result, long-term condition monitoring is required because it is possible for athletes to artificially manipulate biological markers, such as testosterone concentrations (albeit with great difficulty), by taking other substances to gain a beneficial diagnosis, or exceed the therapeutic dosage even if the medical condition is genuine (Di Luigi et al., 2019). At the TUE Committee level, Fitch (2020) recently proposed a WADA accreditation system to ensure a minimum standard of committee that approves applications and bolsters the perceived legitimacy of the TUE process.

Another challenge faced by the TUE process is a lack of research into the specific effects of certain drugs. For example, psychostimulants have been shown to increase athletic performance in healthy populations, but no evidence exists on athletes properly diagnosed with attention deficit hyperactivity disorder (Garner, Hansen, Baxley, & Ross, 2018). Therefore, criteria B in the International Standard for TUE cannot accurately be established. TUE for asthma medication also appears to be stigmatised through its association with cheating; a key activity in addressing the stigma lies with rigorously establishing how asthma medication effects performance (Allen, Backhouse, Hull, & Price, 2019). In response to the criticisms levelled against the TUE system, WADA's TUE group (Gerrard, 2017) published a declaration arguing that the current system is based on consensus between global experts.

The potential use of TUE for performance enhancement has attracted considerable suspicion from athletes (e.g., Bourdon, Schoch, Broers, & Kayser, 2014; Efverström, Ahmadi, Hoff, & Bäckström, 2016; Overbye & Wagner, 2013). Overbye and Wagner (2013) revealed that 46% of athletes who had never been granted a TUE believed athletes get TUEs without a therapeutic need. The percentage increased to 66% for athletes who had previously been granted a TUE. The high percentage of athletes expressing misgivings about the TUE system represents a significant threat to the legitimacy of WADA. Bourdon et al. (2014) also indicated that a significant proportion of athletes avoided seeking treatment due to the potential stigma, given that TUEs are associated with sanctioned doping. A study conducted by WADA in 2020 may go some way to allaying these stigma-based fears, as cross-examination between WADA's TUE database and Olympic performance in individual sports indicated that less than 1% of all athletes competing had a TUE valid at the time of competition, and that there was 'no meaningful association' between TUE athletes and winning an Olympic medal (Vernec & Healy, 2020). Of 2,062 medals awarded across eight Olympic Games, only 21 were won by athletes with an active TUE. We suggest the next step in exploring if there is any relationship between TUE and performance is to examine athletes who have had TUE at other points in their competitive season.

The controversial nature of the TUE system coupled with evidence that some athletes judge it negatively means that the policy provides a unique case in which to explore how different stakeholders have challenged the legitimacy of WADA, and subsequently how WADA has responded. In doing so, this chapter further disassembles the multi-level legitimacy processes around the WADA regime. The following section will outline the specific periods of instability identified in our analysis that led to debate about the TUE system.

Therapeutic use exemptions: key periods of instability

Five key periods emerged in relation to the TUE system that have led to the scrutiny of WADA's legitimacy. The first period occurred during the 2015 Cycling Independent Reform Commission (CIRC) suggesting that the UCI had granted a TUE retrospectively to help Lance Armstrong cover up a positive doping test. Furthermore, the report indicated that the UCI had manipulated the rule for other riders as well (CIRC, 2015). The Commission was financed by the UCI to investigate 'the causes of the pattern of doping that developed within cycling and allegations which implicate the UCI and other governing bodies and officials over ineffective investigation of such practices' (CIRC, 2015, p. 6). When the final report of the commission was published in March 2015, journalists, athletes and members of the anti-doping community used it as an opportunity to criticise the implementation of the TUE rule and WADA. Furthermore, both the UCI and WADA were forced to defend the system (UCI, 2015; WADA, 2015a).

The second period followed allegations that Alberto Salazar, head coach of the Nike-funded 'Oregon Project' for athletics training in the United States, was committing anti-doping rule violations (ADRVs), including misusing the TUE rule. Specifically, in June 2015, a British documentary alleged that Salazar had given testosterone illegally to a 16-year-old athlete and had encouraged athletes to apply for TUE to obtain performance-enhancing benefits. The case generated widespread attention because 5,000-m and 10,000-m world champion Mo Farah was training under Salazar at the time. These allegations stimulated wider debate and criticism of the TUE rule, amongst journalists, athletes and anti-doping experts, as well as generating a public response from WADA (WADA, 2015b). Furthermore, USADA launched an investigation into the Oregon project and the project's affiliated doctor, Jeffrey Brown (Hart, 2017, May 19). It culminated in September 2019 when Salazar received a four-year suspension for ADRVs including administration of a prohibited method (subject to appeal at the time of writing).

The third key period surrounded the announcement of professional tennis player and former world number one Maria Sharapova's positive test for mildronate, also known as meldonium in March 2016. Meldonium was previously a legal medication that was prohibited by WADA at the start of 2016, and therefore required a TUE from this date onwards. Researchers have suggested that when meldonium was a legal substance, it was excessively prescribed in healthy athlete populations contributing to WADA's decision to require a TUE for use (Stuart, Schneider, & Steinbach, 2016). Sharapova failed to obtain a TUE and consequently failed an anti-doping test. Sharapova's position as a former world number one female tennis player meant the jolt generated widespread publicity, intensified by the wider story of the large number of positive tests for meldonium following its ban. Furthermore, journalists and critics raised questions about the therapeutic appropriateness of meldonium in the first place.

The fourth period was associated with the illegal hacking and publication of numerous athlete medical records, including granted TUEs, by the cyber group Fancy Bears. Publication of medical records began in September 2016 and continued until April 2017. Fancy Bears is a cyber-espionage group based in Russia and thought to be linked to the Russian government (Bartlett, 2018, March 26). The data were used by Fancy Bears to allege a double standard between the treatment of Russian athletes associated with the systematic doping programme in Russia before the 2016 Rio de Janeiro Summer Olympics and the number of medallists from other nations who were granted a TUE. Fancy Bears argued that the latter group of athletes were perceived to be cheating within the rules. This was the largest jolt of all the periods mentioned and provoked challenges to the legitimacy of WADA from athletes, journalists and governments. Accordingly, both WADA and countries and sports embroiled in the data leaks responded to safeguard their legitimacy. Furthermore, information published following the data leak raised suspicions about three TUEs granted to British cyclist and Tour de France winner Bradley Wiggins. This motivated the Department for Digital, Culture, Media and Sport (DCMS) in the United Kingdom to investigate if the organisations responsible for Bradley Wiggins, British Cycling and professional cycling team 'Team Sky', followed the correct anti-doping procedures (The Digital, Culture, Media and Sport Select Committee, 2018). The investigation published in March 2018 revealed a legal, but ethically controversial approach to using a TUE for 'marginal gains' in performance. The marginal gains philosophy reflects the idea that small, incremental improvements in all areas of training and preparation leads to significant increased overall performance.

The final period was also related to Team Sky as its lead rider and reigning Tour de France champion at the time, Chris Froome, provided an adverse analytical finding (AAF) during the Vuelta a España race in September 2017. His positive test was later leaked to the public in December 2017. Froome reported twice the permitted limit of salbutamol, a steroid used to treat asthma that can also have performance-enhancing effects. The controversy stemmed from the fact that Froome had been granted a TUE to take salbutamol through an inhaler. Considered in the context of Team Sky's controversial 'marginal gains' policy (The Digital, Culture, Media and Sport Select Committee, 2018), the test result attracted attention from athletes, journalists, anti-doping experts and other teams. In July 2018, the UCI and WADA declared that Froome had been cleared of any wrongdoing and was free to race in the 2018 Tour de France. This decision led many journalists and NADOs to criticise the UCI and WADA's handling of TUEs as well as the lack of transparency in the decision to clear Froome of any wrongdoing.

Tracking the sources and magnitude of the jolts emanating from the five periods, it appears that the first jolt raised debate about TUEs but was limited to journalists, doctors and the UCI. Perhaps, because of its specificity to cycling, the story engaged only sources with a specific interest. Similarly, the second jolt involving Alberto Salazar also generated substantial debate, but mainly between journalists, doctors and anti-doping officials, and it was only the link to Mo Farah that made the jolt more broadly significant. The third and fourth jolts involving Maria Sharapova's positive test and the Fancy Bears leak engaged broader stakeholders in active inspection of WADA's legitimacy. It is at this point that national governments, IFs and professional athletes not directly linked to the jolts began to challenge the legitimacy of WADA on performance grounds increasing the risk to the organisation. Finally, Chris Froome's leaked AAF was arguably a smaller event than the other jolts, but it appears that by this point legitimacy challenges about TUEs had accumulated as stakeholders from outside of cycling used it as an opportunity to challenge WADA. From the legitimacy debates arising around these jolts, three themes consistently emerged from the newspaper data: (1) accuracy of diagnosis, (2) moral ambiguity and (3) political opportunism.

Accuracy of diagnosis

Accuracy of diagnosis reflects the debate that emerged around the importance of doctors in professional sport. Challenges to WADA focused on how the TUE rule is dependent upon the honest diagnosis of medical conditions by medical professionals within sport. If the TUE process can be misused and leads to an unequal playing field, an evaluator may render a negative judgement of the rule. Cox, Bloodworth, and McNamee (2017) commented on the inherent conflict team doctors find themselves in being under pressure to provide medical care and being work-dependent upon the success of the team. Although all TUE applications are examined by an independent TUE committee at the national level and are subject to review by WADA, if the initial information provided to this committee is incorrect, then the rule can be circumvented. Accuracy of diagnosis brings up more specific issues with implementation such as incorrect medical diagnosis, inappropriate treatment of real conditions and retrospective TUE. The issue of correct treatment arises as doctors could deliberately diagnose patients with medical conditions in order to prescribe certain drugs or prescribe unnecessarily strong medication for a genuine ailment. Additionally, the granting of a TUE retrospectively can undermine faith in the system. The capacity to cheat via team doctors challenges the pragmatic legitimacy of WADA in enforcing the TUE rule and providing fair and clean sport to athletes and stakeholders.

Road race cycling and the CIRC report (2015) provided an example of how the theme of accuracy of diagnosis affects WADA's legitimacy. There have been long-term concerns about TUE misuse in cycling, including suggestions that the UCI has actively colluded in misuse (Lawton & Moore, 2013, November 20). In 2015 the CIRC report was published as part of a wider investigation by the UCI into suspicions of doping in cycling. One of the prominent findings from the CIRC report noted that the UCI had previously 'acted in breach of its own anti-doping rules in asking the riders' entourages to provide a medical certificate after they tested positive when they had not declared the use of a substance on the doping control form' (CIRC, 2015, p. 173). Furthermore, the UCI was judged to have broken its anti-doping rules at the 2014 Tour de Romandie in granting British cyclist and Tour de France winner Chris Froome a TUE based on the approval of only one doctor (p. 154). Interviews with a range of stakeholders including but not limited to team staff, UCI and national cycling federation employees, medical practitioners, current and retired cyclists and NADOs suggested that TUE exploitation was ongoing in professional cycling, and one cyclist estimated that 90% of TUEs were for performance enhancement (CIRC, 2015, p. 61). Journalists used the CIRC report to challenge the TUE process (e.g., Dickinson, 2015, March 9; Fotheringham, 2015, March 9; Gibson, 2015, March 12). For example, UK journalist Matt Dickinson (2015, March 9) argued: 'More than anything, they [fans] want to know if they can trust the sport now and, on this key issue, the CIRC report is as troubling as it is reassuring'. Statements like this capture the feeling that the TUE process undermined the legitimacy of WADA to achieve its purpose of helping keep sport doping free.

Accuracy of diagnosis was also a theme during the Oregon Project allegations, as it was alleged Alberto Salazar had encouraged his athletes to seek medical prescriptions to help reduce fatigue and lose weight. The deliberate attempt to gain advantages through misdiagnosis highlighted the role of doctors in doping (Daly & Epstein, 2017, May 30). The Oregon Project case demonstrated the conflict doctors can face between providing medical care to athletes as well as supporting the team. The long-term consequences of incorrect diagnosis have resulted in one former Oregon Project athlete being left dependent on the medication thyroxanol, as drug misuse has altered the athlete's natural hormonal system (Al-Samarrai & Hughes, 2019). Correspondingly, Maria Sharapova's positive test for the anti-ischemic medication (i.e., used to prevent and treat heart disease) meldonium, thought to potentially improve endurance, centred on the accuracy of diagnosis. Her use generated criticisms from journalists to the TUE rule because of the appropriateness of meldonium as (1) she had been using it periodically for 10 years, yet, recommended usage was four to six weeks, and (2) it was not approved by the Food and Drug Administration in the United States where she trained (Cambers, 2016, March 10).

Accuracy of diagnosis was also a key theme of the legitimacy debate emerging after Fancy Bears leaked athlete medical information. Journalists raised concerns about the appropriateness of the TUEs granted as high-profile Olympic medallists with TUE were revealed. Although no wrongdoing was directly claimed, some observers remained sceptical. Australian journalist David Moase (2016, September 28) wrote:

> After years of having our faith in the integrity of sport stretched by drug takers, certain athletes are having to answer difficult questions about the medications they have been permitted to use and whether those drugs were more performance enhancing than therapeutic.

Moase's fears were not alleviated by the investigation into Team Sky which uncovered that team doctor Richard Freeman had failed to keep an accurate record of TUEs granted, as well as suspicious timing of the TUEs for cyclist Wiggins who 'was granted TUEs to use the powerful corticosteroid triamcinolone before his three biggest races in 2011, 2012 and 2013, including his famous 2012 Tour de France victory' (Associated Press, 2016, December 18). The jolt generated criticisms from a range of stakeholders as it coupled with former Team Sky coach Shane Sutton's comments about TUEs 'that finding the gains might mean getting a TUE? Yes, because the rules allow you to do that' ('Sutton defends', 2017, November 18). For example, sport law professor Jack Anderson remarked: 'The TUE process has long provoked disquiet as to how some of the fittest people on the planet appear, paradoxically, to need extensive medication for underlying conditions'. Other sources targeted WADA directly. For example, the DCMS Committee (2018) called on WADA to ban all corticosteroids after receiving evidence that they could be misused through the TUE rule. Floyd Landis, a former Tour De France winner, stripped of his title for doping declared:

> I can't see how the sport authorities can let it slide. You can't take them seriously if they don't act. There's a report right there for them and for me WADA have no choice but to suspend him [Bradley Wiggins] and take his title away. If they were legitimate, that's what they'd do.
>
> (Cary, 2018, March 6)

Although there is no evidence of an ADRV, these comments reflect an attitude that the TUE process has failed to deliver clean sport as part of WADA's mission and may have in fact increased drug use in sport. The TUE process is not providing benefits to athletes who are not using a TUE or other sources who depend upon sport being clean.

WADA's position has remained one of defiance (Oliver, 1991) in dismissing challenges arising concerning accuracy of diagnosis. For example, in June 2014, the French newspaper *Journal du Dimanche* claimed that the UCI had incorrectly granted Chris Froome a TUE for a corticosteroid by not making the application subject to a committee review (Whittle, 2014, June 17). A WADA press statement specified, however, that it was satisfied with the decision by the UCI and did not pursue the case further (Whittle, 2014, June 17). In contrast, the UCI declared that it would be 'reviewing all of its anti-doping rules and procedures including those regarding Therapeutic Use Exemptions' (Cary, 2014, June 24). Later, when the same accusations emerged after the CIRC report was published, WADA President Sir Craig Reedie commented generally on the TUE rule: 'We monitor this system carefully to make sure that people don't try to abuse it for their own gain. You can always look at tightening up such systems but we are satisfied that the rules are strong' (Reedie, 2015). Following the release of the DCMS (2018) report, WADA dismissed the findings and did not provide comment (Kelner, 2018, March 5). WADA's decision defied logic given the high-profile nature of the criticism and the UCI's decision to investigate corticosteroid use based on the report findings and eventual decision to ban the substance.

WADA also dismissed challenges arising from the Fancy Bears leak. In a WADA press release in response to the Fancy Bears data leaks, the TUE Expert Group stated: 'The WADA TUE Expert Group confirms its unequivocal support for the existing process by which athletes with genuine medical conditions may obtain appropriate clinical care and remain active in sport' (WADA, 2016a). Again, WADA was confident in dismissing legitimacy challenges. Other organisations challenged by the leaked data adopted this defiant approach, arguing that the system was sound. The USADA Chief Executive Travis Tygart remarked: 'The truth is, it would be foolish to try to cheat this way. If you're trying to cheat, the idea that you would self-disclose what you're already using, or want to use that is illegal, isn't very bright' (Litke, 2016, September 20).

WADA's defiant approach in response to challenges aligns with the tenets of multi-level legitimacy theory. The media are recognised sources of legitimacy. If WADA were to capitulate or compromise in response to external challenges, it would suggest an admission of fault, and perhaps, negligence. It may be that in highly contested fields where an organisation's legitimacy rests on a weak consensus of validity, acknowledging fault and/or acquiescing to challenges opens the potential for fierce debate and evaluation from suppressed stakeholders. Indeed, without a confession or direct evidence of dishonest behaviour in the TUE process, it is exceptionally difficult to determine if the TUE process has been manipulated (Cox et al., 2017).

Moral ambiguity

The second point emerging from legitimacy debates about the TUE system is moral ambiguity, which captures arguments about (1) whether TUE should be allowed at all and, if so, (2) how transparent its use should be. This is different from accuracy of diagnosis as it challenges the legitimacy of the TUE rule about whether it is acceptable by moral criteria rather than if the system can be misused. There is a moral debate between those who believe athletes should have the right to medical treatment during competition (e.g., WADA), and critics who believe athletes who require medical treatment (that may have a performance-enhancing effect) should be forced to stop competing temporarily. In certain cases, such as asthma or attention deficit hyperactivity disorder that require lifelong treatment, discarding TUE exemptions would mean permanent exclusion from professional sport or living without medication to compete. By implication, a moral legitimacy judgement arises as to whether athletes should be allowed to simultaneously take potentially performance-enhancing medicine and compete. Furthermore, with the knowledge that inaccurate diagnoses could undermine the TUE rule, critics have suggested increasing transparency in the TUE process to deter malfeasance, for example, by publishing all TUE applications. These negative judgements undermine the legitimacy of WADA in the correct way to manage drugs in sport.

Challenges around the moral ambiguity of TUE vary in severity. Suggestions have ranged from completely abandoning the TUE rule, banning participation if an athlete is currently using a TUE substance (Williams, 2016, September 23) or declaring which athletes have a TUE but not what they are for (Axon, 2016, September 20). Following the CIRC report and the failings of the TUE procedure, journalist Paul Kimmage proclaimed: 'The only thing that can save this sport is transparency' (Kimmage, 2015, July 19). The Fancy Bears data leak also led to arguments for increased transparency in the TUE process because commentators questioned why so many elite athletes required a TUE (Ziegler, 2016, September 15). For example, journalist Scott Wilson argued: 'While there is an understandable concern about breaching medical confidentiality, athletes applying for a TUE should have to agree that if it is granted, it will become public knowledge. No hidden files; no uncertainty about who is taking what' (Wilson, 2016, September 23). Jonathan Vaughters, Chief Executive of the Cannondale-Drapac cycling team similarly argued for transparency: 'Any athlete would think twice unless they really needed it' (Williams, 2016, September 23). Certain athletes have also argued they would be happy to provide TUE data (Van Royen, 2016, October 5). Yet, for every moral judgement that reasoned for transparency, NADOs and WADA argued against increased transparency. For example, Nicole Sapstead (2016), Chief Executive Officer of UKAD, contended:

If athletes want to put that information out there, they are perfectly entitled to. But as far as we are concerned, this is confidential medical data - often for deeply personal conditions - which we are committed to protecting. Even publishing redacted TUE is problematic because, without the proper context, people can jump to the wrong conclusion.

Furthermore, WADA Executive Committee meeting minutes revealed that despite negative attention from the press, the Executive Committee had faith in the TUE rule (WADA, 2016b). However, changes made in relation to the Fancy Bears hack included increasing digital security to prevent further hacking, rather than improving the process itself (WADA, 2017).

Suggestions about more draconian TUE rules prohibiting participation were advocated, such as the following proposed by sport scientist Ross Tucker:

I would consider banning all TUE in competition. I know it is a hard-line stance. But what would be the downside if people with asthma cannot compete? Conceptually to me, that is fine. Because unfortunately the efforts to be inclusive with people who have valid medical issues have created a loophole that is being exploited by sophisticated dopers.

(Menon, 2016)

Equally, journalists have debated the merits of banning the use of TUE in professional sport when considering the case of Chris Froome and Fancy Bears (Dickinson, 2016, September 20; Williams, 2016, September 23). Others have proposed less severe measures. For example, British doctor John Dickinson, a specialist in exercise-induced asthma and Team GB employee, suggested that there could be a temporary suspension from competition (e.g., two weeks) following treatment using certain substances such as corticosteroids (Majendie, 2016, September 20).

Moral arguments about losing the right to medical treatment whilst remaining in professional sport were also ignored by WADA. Defiance is expected when internal organisational values do not match external expectations. Anti-doping is meant to protect athletes, however, removing the right to medical treatment only further victimises the athlete. Therefore, WADA and other anti-doping officials had no choice but to stand behind the current TUE process. For example, in response to the release of medical data on Australian swimmers, Chief Medical Officer for Australian Swimming Peter Fricker said:

The TUE process exists because we want people to be able to compete and to have medical treatment if there is a valid health reason and they need the treatment. It's designed so that we can use appropriate treatment for medical conditions.

(Jeffery, 2016, October 5)

The sentiment that athletes are entitled to treatment and that the rules will not change was echoed by other anti-doping officials (Axon, 2016, September 20), including David Gerrard, head of WADA's TUE Committee: 'Although we do have some concerns about the consistency in some parts of the world, the major players in the rest of the world have robust TUE committees and rigorously support and endorse the processes that are in place' (Van Royen, 2016, October 5). The TUE Committee's observations further indicated faith in the current process allowing athletes the right to privacy and medical treatment. This stance was consistent across statements from other WADA officials ('WADA defends TUE system', 2016, September 28). Defiance may stem from the fact that the current TUE process is the only workable policy available to WADA. For example, sport lawyer and former Olympian Alex Kelham highlighted the problem that increasing transparency in the TUE process has the potential to tarnish an athlete's reputation by association. Concerning Chris Froome's clearance of any wrongdoing, she asserted: 'The media could adopt the line that therapeutic use exemptions make sport possible for thousands of people who would not be able to compete otherwise and therefore should not be frowned on' (Ames, 2018, July 5).

It is worth noting the single instance in which WADA appeared to compromise to a growing challenge before withdrawing its response. The DCMS (2018) review brought Bradley Wiggins' use of Triamcinolone, a corticosteroid with potential performance-enhancing effects also used for the treatment of asthma and allergies, under scrutiny. A week later, WADA Director General Olivier Niggli stated in reference to TUE for glucosteroids that 'it is an unsatisfactory situation, we all agree with that. And we have set up a group to try to come up with better proposal to how we can do it' (Ziegler, 2017 March 8). WADA's Health, Medical and Research Committee later discussed the problems with glucosteroids citing that it is still impossible to determine if they were administered legally (WADA, 2017). Later in March 2018, when the DCMS report concluded:

> The TUE system needs to be kept under permanent review, but the question inevitably remains, that if an athlete is so ill that they can only compete using a drug that is otherwise banned during competition, then why are they competing at all?
>
> (DCMS, 2018, p. 31)

The report went further, explicitly stating that WADA should ban all use of glucocorticoids (p. 32). Following these conclusions challenging athlete's rights to treatment, WADA failed to provide any official response to the investigation. It constituted a change in stance by ignoring the challenges, despite having previously stated that it would investigate glucosteroid use.

WADA's response to individuals who had questioned the moral ambiguity of TUE such as the accuracy of diagnosis, was one of defiance. Such defiance in the face of moral challenges may be better understood in light of WADA's justification for taking a prohibitive approach to anti-doping policy. Although it could be argued that the current prohibition approach does not protect health (cf. Møller, 2016), anti-doping is built upon the premise that doping prohibition policies are designed to protect athlete welfare. Therefore, to renege on this point would undermine the philosophy of the current prohibition system. WADA could not maintain a stance that TUEs are not allowed, and simultaneously argue that one of their primary purposes is to promote athlete welfare.

Prohibitive anti-doping policy is founded upon the amateur notions of performance enhancement being contrary to the spirit of sport. In this case, it appears that WADA finds itself in a paradoxical position where it must defy criticism about the TUE process to maintain its discourse around protecting athlete welfare, while simultaneously maintaining regulations that cannot accurately measure the extent to which individuals experience performance enhancement (Pike, 2018). The contradiction was described as corrupt idealism by Møller (2014), as shortcomings in anti-doping implementation are permitted so as not to undermine the overall objective and philosophy.

Political opportunism

The final theme to emerge from legitimacy debates about the TUE rule is termed *political opportunism*, which reflects how stakeholders used perceived shortcomings in the TUE rule to challenge WADA's fitness to regulate anti-doping. WADA has previously been criticised for being euro-centric, dividing the global north and south as well as promoting moral values on behalf of the IOC. As a result, despite being a global organisation, WADA is dominated by Western European, North American and Antipodean political views. This scepticism mirrors the historical influence of the Cold War that influenced anti-doping in the 1970s and 1980s (Hunt, 2011). The debate around the TUE rule revealed that certain groups held suppressed judgements about the legitimacy of WADA as a regulatory body. During the periods following scandals, stakeholders may seek to challenge the assumption that WADA is the only organisation capable of managing anti-doping.

The problem of meldonium exemplifies the issue of political opportunism. Meldonium is manufactured in Latvia and was created as an anti-ischemic medication for Soviet Forces fighting at altitude (Rumsby, 2016, March 9). Consequently, it was predominantly prescribed in Eastern European countries, and the majority of the 60 positive tests within the first 10 weeks of prohibition were Eastern European and Russian athletes (Dickinson, 2016, March 9). However, the decision to make meldonium a prohibited substance was problematic due to a lack of data about how long meldonium remained present in urine. The wave of positive tests generated a reaction from Russian officials (Walker, 2016, March 8), including Russian President Vladimir Putin, who defended Russian athletes: 'This substance was never considered as doping. It doesn't influence the result. That's totally certain. It just keeps the heart muscles in good condition under high load' (Associated Press, 2016). The realisation that no data had been collected on the excretion time of meldonium provided Russian officials with an opportunity to challenge the legitimacy of WADA, arguing that doping was 'being used as a political weapon against Russia' (Grove, 2016, March 11). WADA was characteristically defiant in response to these challenges, and maintained that the prohibition decision was evidence based. The statement by David Howman, WADA Director General, reinforced WADA's position:

> The reason for it being on the list is it's being used and has been used to enhance people's performance, and that was the reason for this substance first to be monitored for 12 months. There was ample warning, if you like, given when it was put on the monitoring list in 2014 for people to say, 'Hey, we have to be careful here' and they weren't.
>
> (Clarey, 2016, March 10)

WADA did, however, accept certain aspects of the arguments made by Russian officials and undertook further research into the excretion time of meldonium, eventually conceding that test results under one microgram per millilitre taken within 12 weeks of meldonium being banned could be deemed 'no fault' (WADA, 2016c). Although WADA was quick to state that the change 'should not be seen as an amnesty for athletes' (Reveell, 2016, April 13), the situation demonstrated how suppressed groups can use challenges to create more favourable conditions; in this instance, the ability for Russia to contest WADA's decision to ban meldonium.

Russia continued to challenge the legitimacy of WADA following the Fancy Bears data leak. Russian TV portrayed WADA as permissive of doping in certain countries (BBC, 2016), and the Russian embassy tweeted about the perceived double standard between Russian and American athletes (Ziegler, 2016, September 15). Like he did in the meldonium example, Vladimir Putin commented on the use of TUE in Western athletes contending, 'Maybe they can be put in a special category, or their achievements, points, seconds and honours can be considered in a special way' (Berry, 2016, October 12). The propriety judgements of Russian media and officials assumed that Russian athletes had been unfairly treated by WADA compared to Western athletes. This has been linked to an attempt to discredit the damage done by the exposure of systematic doping (Kelly, 2016, September 20). Interestingly though, other nations that have been criticised by WADA and associated with doping also took advantage of the data leak. For example, Indian journalist Suresh Menon wrote critically of the TUE rule:

> WADA cannot be unaware of the manner in which the TUE can be misused. Given that, the body is either incompetent or complicit, and neither is acceptable. I suspect too that not enough is known about the performance-enhancing qualities of drugs used medically.
>
> (Menon, 2016)

It is noteworthy that India had the sixth-highest number of ADRV in the world in 2016 (WADA, 2018a). Correspondingly, Ethiopia has been reprimanded by WADA due to concerns about the prevalence of doping in the country (Meseret, 2016, April 7), and the Ethiopian press pointed out the double standards. For example, an article published in the state-owned newspaper *Ethiopian Herald* criticised the TUE rule and Western athletes, implying WADA's complicity in allowing athletes from selected nations to cheat:

> The intriguing aspect is that WADA currently defends the cheats. No one dares to resign from global anti-doping office for this. In the true sense of the legal aspect, they (the WADA officials) have to be punished for their double standard medical report.
>
> ('WADA's fight', 2016)

The previous quotes imply a shared propriety judgement that WADA was biased against certain nations. Moreover, it suggests an attempt by those individuals and organisations who are suppressed and have an unfavourable institutional environment to challenge the very existence of WADA by questioning its biases. There was merit in the challenges as they highlighted the system can be misused. However, their legitimacy as a stakeholder to challenge WADA appears to be lacking and was easily dismissed, as seen in WADA's responses.

Implicated nations, organisations and WADA were defiant against accusations of wrongdoing, arguing that all TUEs had been granted through the correct procedure. For example, WADA's senior science director Olivier Rabin voiced WADA's view that 'TUEs fall under international standards. They are scrutinised by the medical community' ('Agency defends', 2016, September 29). Likewise, the British Triathlon Federation defended its athletes: 'Let's be very clear; athletes who have a TUE on their record have followed the rules based on a specific medical requirement. We can say with absolute confidence that our athletes have nothing to hide' (Phillips, 2016, October 3). Other organisations followed the same line of defiance grounded in adherence with the TUE process. For example, Canada Soccer defended its implicated athletes: 'Canada Soccer carefully followed the appropriate procedures to allow for the use of these medications by our athletes' (Kelly, 2016, September 20).

There is an interesting contrast in the language chosen by those challenging and defending the TUE system. Challengers typically used the term *performance-enhancing substance*, whereas defenders referred to *medication and medical requirements*. It may be that challengers utilised this terminology to infer negative judgements about the legitimacy of the TUE process to other stakeholders, while defenders chose the term *medication* to legitimise the TUE process through association with the scientific legitimacy of medicine.

Consistent with WADA's response to other legitimacy challenges related to TUE, there was typically an unwillingness to accept any fault, and responsibility was displaced by asserting adherence to the rules. Their argument was that because they followed the rules there was no fault. Yet, WADA had determined the rules, and this argument does not satisfy the criticisms raised about the dependence on honest and accurate diagnoses by medical professionals working for sports teams. Journalist Kevin Ferrie summed this up:

> The British are lauded because everything they [British Athletics] have done has been within the rules. The Russians are meanwhile ostracised. Is it morally wrong to wonder how the rule book might read if it was initially published in Cyrillic rather than English?
>
> (Ferrie, 2016, September 22)

Finally, political opportunism was evident following the case of Chris Froome. Chris Froome was cleared of wrongdoing by the UCI, a decision supported by WADA (WADA, 2018b; UCI, 2018). However, the decision was met with scepticism from cyclists and French newspapers who challenged the legitimacy of the decision by arguing that WADA was scared of a costly legal battle with Froome as well as questioning whether WADA was the right organisation to tackle anti-doping (Fotheringham, 2018, July 3). In a rare response of acquiescence, WADA provided further details of the case, responding to challenges from multiple stakeholders arguing that the maximum limit set for a salbutamol TUE was appropriate and there were exceptional circumstances around Froome's test result (WADA, 2018c). However, the response failed to settle the challenges to WADA as journalists questioned why a pharmacokinetic study (an analysis of drug absorption and metabolism rates) was not necessary when other salbutamol cases had required them (Whittle, 2018, July 12). The lack of transparency in Froome's case has been used to directly challenge the assumption that WADA should regulate anti-doping. Head of USADA Travis Tygart queried: 'The question is whether justice was truly served or did a star get an undeserved break. Unfortunately, it's another blow to the perceived credibility of the global anti-doping movement' (Nathanson & Skelton, 2018, July 25). The United States has been critical of WADA since its inception due to the perceived conflict of interest with the IOC (as noted in chapter three). USADA leveraged the handling of Chris Froome's case to further its own judgement. WADA responded to Tygart by dismissing his claims as 'uninformed, unconstructive, and, quite frankly is surprising' (Nathanson & Skelton, 2018, July 25).

It could be argued that the human right to medical treatment exceeds all legitimacy challenges, despite the potential for exploitation. However, it could also be contended that the sources of the legitimacy challenges possessed little influence. We argue that the value of being perceived as legitimate by select journalists, individual experts and reprimanded nations was of little consideration to WADA. A comment from Sir Craig Reedie during the Fancy Bears leak is telling in this regard: 'We will have to wait to see whether there's sufficient demand from stakeholders to review what we do' (Majendie, 2016,

September 16). Until an influential group of stakeholders launches a sustained challenge against the TUE process, there is little motivation for WADA to re-evaluate the policy. Therefore, defiance may be part of a larger discourse to maintain the institutionalised relationships between organisations in the field of anti-doping. In this regard, research suggesting that WADA is an external arm of the IOC's influence in sport is relevant (Dimeo & Møller, 2018). Acquiescing or compromising to beliefs challenging WADA would be detrimental to the groups which currently benefit from the current arrangement.

Conclusion

In conclusion, the discussion of the TUE process has revolved around accuracy of diagnosis, moral ambiguity and political opportunism. Our analysis points to differing beliefs about WADA which formed varying levels of legitimacy challenges. We have described how certain sources expressed negative beliefs about the TUE system's pragmatic and moral legitimacy. The TUE system's lack of legitimacy has been used to challenge WADA's impartiality and objectivity. Accordingly, the TUE process currently represents a threat to the existence of WADA should scandals continue to occur involving TUE misuse. WADA's response to these challenges has been characterised by defiance, which is explained by two primary points: (1) WADA cannot simultaneously justify anti-doping by protecting athlete welfare and then not allow them medical treatment and (2) to yield to these challenges meant WADA risked drawing further scrutiny and evaluation of the discourses it has created around being a global organisation protecting athlete welfare. In the broader discussion of WADA's legitimacy, these conclusions support an emerging picture of WADA's reliance on a defiant approach to responding to legitimacy challenges. From a theoretical perspective, we argue that the legitimacy of a challenger, as in the previous chapters, appears as important as the content of a legitimacy challenge. In the next chapter, we present a discussion of the investigation into the use of performance-enhancing drugs by Australian Football League side, Essendon Football Club. In this chapter, we have witnessed how anti-doping scandals can lead to legitimacy challenges for WADA policy. Extending our analysis further, the Essendon Football Club case demonstrates how poor governance and regulation of sport can create connected legitimacy challenges between teams, anti-doping organisations and WADA.

References

Agency defends therapeutic drug exemptions (2016, September 29). *The Mercury*. Retrieved from https://www.iol.co.za/mercury.

Allen, H., Backhouse, S.H., Hull, J.H., & Price, O.J. (2019). Anti-doping policy, therapeutic use exemption and medication use in athletes with asthma: A narrative review and critical appraisal of current regulations. *Sports Medicine*, 49(5), 659–668.

Al-Samarrai, R. & Hughes, M. (2019). UK Athletics drug claims: British stars say governing body encouraged legal use of thyroid medication to enhance performance, as top athletes fear spread of the dubious methods used by Mo Farah's ex coach Alberto Salazar. *The Daily Mail*. Retrieved from https://www.dailymail.co.uk/.

Ames, J. (2018, July 5). The race to restore a reputation. Retrieved from https://www.thetimes.co.uk.

Associated Press. (2016, December 18). Brailsford to be asked 'important questions' says sports minister. *The Daily Mail*.

Axon, R. (2016, September 20). Records hack shows flaws. *USA Today*. Retrieved from https://www.usatoday.com.

Bartlett, E. (2018 March 26). Fancy Bears: Who are the shady hacking group exposing doping, cover-ups and corruption in sport? *The Independent*. Retrieved from https://www.independent.co.uk/.

BBC. (2016, September 19). Russian TV weekly highlights: Duma election, spat with US over Syria, doping row. *The BBC*. Retrieved from https://monitoring.bbc.co.uk/.

Berry, J. (2016, October 12). Putin's call to ban all TUE athletes laughable, says anti-doping body. *The Irish Daily Mail*.

Bourdon, F., Schoch, L., Broers, B., & Kayser, B. (2014). French speaking athletes' experience and perception regarding the whereabouts reporting system and therapeutic use exemptions. *Performance Enhancement & Health*, 3(3–4), 153–158.

Cambers, S. (2016, March 10). Why was Maria Sharapova taking meldonium? *The Guardian*. Retrieved from https://www.theguardian.com/uk 219.

Cary, T. (2014, June 24). Froome case prompts new TUE process. *The Daily Telegraph*. Retrieved from https://www.telegraph.co.uk.

Cary, T. (2018, March 6). Team Sky will not be at the Tour de France this year, predicts Floyd Landis. *The Telegraph*. Retrieved from https://www.telegraph.co.uk/.

CIRC. (2015). Report to the president of the Union Cycliste Internationale. *Cycling Independent Reform Commission*. Lausanne, Switzerland.

Clarey, C. (2016, March 10). More than 60 athletes have tested positive for meldonium. *The New York Times*. Retrieved from https://www.nytimes.com.

Cox, L., Bloodworth, A., & McNamee, M. (2017). Olympic doping, transparency, and the therapeutic exemption process. *Diagoras: International Academic Journal on Olympic Studies*, 1, 55–74.

Daly, M., & Epstein, D. (2017, May 30). Drug probe doctor 'altered athlete medical records'. BBC. Retrieved from https://www.bbc.co.uk/.

Di Luigi, L., Pigozzi, F., Sgrò, P., Frati, L., Di Gianfrancesco, A., & Cappa, M. (2019). The use of prohibited substances for therapeutic reasons in athletes affected by endocrine diseases and disorders: the therapeutic use exemption (TUE) in clinical endocrinology. *Journal of Endocrinological Investigation*, 43, 563–573. 10.1007/s40618-019-01145-z.

Dickinson, M. (2015, March 9). Doping war reveals old habits die hard. *The Times*. Retrieved from http://www.thetimes.co.uk.

Dickinson, M. (2016, March 9). Meldonium: The 'poor man's EPO' with 60 positive tests in ten weeks. *The Times*. Retrieved from http://www.thetimes.co.uk.

The Digital, Culture, Media and Sport Select Committee. (2018). Combatting doping in sport. Retrieved from https://www.gov.uk/government/organisations/department-for-digital-culture-media-sport.

Dimeo, P., & Møller, V. (2018). *The Anti-Doping Crisis in Sport*. London, UK: Routledge 10.4324/9781315545677.

Efverström, A., Ahmadi, N., Hoff, D., & Bäckström, Å. (2016). Anti-doping and legitimacy: an international survey of elite athletes' perceptions. *International Journal of Sport Policy and Politics*, 8(3), 491–514.

Ferrie, K. (2016, September 22). How bad is elite sport for your health? Evidence is disturbing. *The Herald*. Retrieved from http://www.heraldscotland.com/.

Fitch, K. (2013). Therapeutic use exemptions (TUEs) at the Olympic Games 1992–2012. *British Journal of Sports Medicine*, 47, 815–818.

Fitch, K. (2020). Therapeutic Use Exemptions (TUEs) are essential in sport: But there is room for improvement. *British Journal of Sports Medicine*, 54(3), 191–192.

Fotheringham, W. (2015, March 9). Lance Armstrong and UCI 'colluded to bypass doping accusations'. *The Guardian*. Retrieved from https://www.theguardian.com/uk.

Fotheringham, W. (2018, July 3). Wada head of science unconcerned about fallout from Chris Froome case. *The Guardian*. Retrieved from https://www.theguardian.com/sport/2018/jul/03/chris-froome-team-sky-leader-tour-de-france.

Garner, A.A., Hansen, A.A., Baxley, C., & Ross, M.J. (2018). The use of stimulant medication to treat attention-deficit/hyperactivity disorder in elite athletes: A performance and health perspective. *Sports Medicine*, 48(3), 507–512.

Gerrard, D. (2017). The use and abuse of the therapeutic use exemptions process. *Current sports medicine reports*, 16(5), 370.

Gibson, O. (2015, March 12). Nicole Cooke criticises UCI over Chris Froome steroid use at Tour of Romandie. *The Guardian*. Retrieved from https://www.theguardian.com/uk.

Grove, T. (2016, March 11). Russia's sports minister accepts some responsibility for meldonium scandal. *The Wall Street Journal*. Retrieved from https://www.wsj.com.

Hart, M. (2017, May 19). 'This doesn't sound legal': Inside Nike's Oregon Project. *The New York Times*. Retrieved from https://www.nytimes.com/.

Hughes, D., Vlahovich, N., Welvaert, M., Tee, N., Harcourt, P., White, S. ... & Waddington, G. (2020). Glucocorticoid prescribing habits of sports medicine physicians working in high-performance sport: A 30-nation survey. *British Journal of Sports Medicine*, 54(7), 402–407.

Hunt, T.M. (2011). *Drug games: The International Olympic Committee and the politics of doping, 1960–2008*. Austin, TX: University of Texas Press.

Jeffery, N. (2016, October 5) Seebohm victim of Fancy Bears. *The Australian*. Retrieved from https://www.theaustralian.com.au/.

Kelly, C. (2016, September 20). Drug use was 'approved by medical committees'. *The Globe and Mail*. Retrieved from https://www.theglobeandmail.com/.

Kelner, M. (2018 March 5). Wiggins case adds to concerns over TUEs, says cycling's governing body. *The Guardian*. Retrieved from www.theguardian.com.

Kimmage, P. (2015, July 19). All we need is transparency. *The Independent*. Retrieved from https://www.independent.co.uk/.

Lawton, M., & Moore, R. (2013, November 20). Cycling chief: I spoke to lance. *The Daily Mail*. Retrieved from http://www.dailymail.co.uk.

Lentillon-Kaestner, V., Hagger, M.S., & Hardcastle, S. (2012). Health and doping in elite-level cycling. *Scandinavian Journal of Medicine & Science in Sports*, 22(5), 596–606.

Litke, J. (2016, September 20). 5 from U.S. had OKs for drugs. *Dayton Daily News*. Retrieved from https://www.daytondailynews.com/.

Majendie, M. (2016, September 16). Anti-doping chiefs to discuss 'abuse' of TUEs. *The Evening Standard*. Retrieved from https://www.standard.co.uk.

Menon, S. (2016). WADA hacking shows up hypocrisy, sets off a necessary debate. *The Hindu*. Retrieved from http://www.thehindu.com/.

Meseret, E. (2016, April 7) Ethiopia told to do mass doping tests or face IAAF ban. *Ethiosports*. Retrieved from http://www.ethiosports.com.

Moase, D. (2016, September 28). Bears put scare in sports. *The Daily Examiner*. Retrieved from https://www.dailyexaminer.com.au/.

Møller, V. (2014). Who guards the guardians?. *The International Journal of the History of Sport, 31*(8), 934–950.

Møller, V. (2016). The road to hell is paved with good intentions—A critical evaluation of WADA's anti-doping campaign. *Performance Enhancement & Health, 4*(3–4), 111–115.

Nathanson, P., & Skelton. J. (2018, July 25). Chris Froome case is a 'blow' to WADA's credibility - USADA head Travis Tygart. *BBC*. Retrieved from https://www.bbc.co.uk/sport/cycling/44924435.

Oliver, C. (1991). Strategic responses to institutional processes. *Academy of Management Review, 16*(1), 145–179.

Overbye, M., & Wagner, U. (2013). Between medical treatment and performance enhancement: An investigation of how elite athletes experience therapeutic use exemptions. *International Journal of Drug Policy, 24*(6), 579–588.

Phillips, M. (2016, October 3). Triathlete Alistair Brownlee laughs off TUE leak. *Channel News Asia*. Retrieved from https://www.uk.reuters.com.

Pike, J. (2018). Therapeutic use exemptions and the doctrine of double effect. *Journal of the Philosophy of Sport, 45*(1), 68–82.

Pitsiladis, Y., Wang, G., Lacoste, A., Schneider, C., Smith, A.D., Di Gianfrancesco, A. & Pigozzi, F. (2017). Make sport great again: the use and abuse of the therapeutic use exemptions process. *Current Sports Medicine Reports, 16*(3), 123–125.

Reedie, C. (2015, July 9). Our rules are strong enough to stop the dopers cheating. *The Independent*. Retrieved from https://www.independent.co.uk/.

Reveell, P. (2016). WADA opens a door for athletes who tested positive for meldonium. *The New York Times*. Retrieved from https://www.nytimes.com.

Rumsby, B. (2016, March 9). How the odds are stacked up against the Russian. *The Daily Telegraph*. Retrieved from https://www.telegraph.co.uk.

Sapstead, N. (2016, September 25) Controversy over TUEs can only lead to better future and instil more confidence. *The Daily Telegraph*. Retrieved from https://www.telegraph.co.uk.

Selge, C., Thomas, S., Nowak, D., Radon, K., & Wolfarth, B. (2016). Asthma prevalence in German Olympic athletes: A comparison of winter and summer sport disciplines. *Respiratory Medicine, 118*, 15–21.

Stuart, M., Schneider, C., & Steinbach, K. (2016). Meldonium use by athletes at the Baku 2015 European Games. *British Journal of Sports Medicine, 50*(11), 694–698.

Sutton defends Wiggins' TUE use for marginal gains. (2017, November 18). *Cycling News*. Retrieved from http://www.cyclingnews.com/.

UCI. (2015). 2015 End of year update - Brian Cookson, President of the Union Cycliste Internationale - Part 1. Retrieved from http://www.uci.ch/.

UCI. (2018). UCI statement on anti-doping proceedings involving Mr Christopher Froome. Retrieved from http://www.uci.ch/pressreleases/uci-statement-anti-doping-proceedings-involving-christopher-froome/.

Van Royen, R. (2016, October 5). Gerrard blasts Russian hackers for leaks. *The Dominion Post*. Retrieved from https://www.stuff.co.nz/dominion-post/.

Vernec, A., & Healy, D. (2020). Prevalence of therapeutic use exemptions at the Olympic Games and association with medals: An analysis of data from 2010 to 2018. *British Journal of Sports Medicine*, 54(15). 10.1136/bjsports-2020-102028.

WADA. (2015a). WADA director general statement on the Cycling Independent Reform Commission. Retrieved from https://www.wada-ama.org/.

WADA. (2015b). WADA statement on BBC panorama programme. Retrieved from https://www.wada-ama.org/en/.

WADA. (2016a). Independent opinion from WADA's TUE Expert Group. Retrieved from https://www.wada-ama.org/.

WADA. (2016b). Minutes of the WADA Executive Committee meeting November 19, 2016, Glasgow, UK. Retrieved from https://www.wada-ama.org.

WADA. (2016c). WADA issues updated Stakeholder guidance regarding meldonium. Retrieved from https://www.wada-ama.org.

WADA. (2017). Minutes of the WADA Executive Committee meeting, May 17, 2017, Montreal, Canada. Retrieved from https://www.wada-ama.org.

WADA. (2018a). 2016 Anti-doping rule violations (ADRVs) report. Retrieved from https://www.wada-ama.org.

WADA. (2018b). WADA will not appeal UCI decision in Christopher Froome case. Retrieved from https://www.wada-ama.org/en/media/news/2018-07/wada-will-not-appeal-uci-decision-in-christopher-froome-case.

WADA. (2018c). WADA clarifies facts regarding UCI decision on Christopher Froome. Retrieved from https://www.wada-ama.org/en/media/news/2018-07/wada-clarifies-facts-regarding-uci-decision-on-christopher-froome.

WADA. (2020). International Standard for Therapeutic Use Exemptions. Retrieved from https://www.wada-ama.org.

WADA defends TUE system. (2016, September 28). *Reuters*. Retrieved from https://uk.reuters.com/.

Wada's fight to insure clean athletes becomes double standard (2016, October 18). *The Ethiopian Herald*. Retrieved from https://www.ethpress.gov.et.

WADC. (2020). World Anti-Doping Code 2021. https://www.wada-ama.org/.

Walker, S. (2016, March 8). Russians warn more athletes could test for Maria Sharapova drug meldonium. *The Guardian*. Retrieved from https://www.theguardian.com/.

Whittle, J. (2014 June 17). Anti-doping agency happy with UCI over Froome's exemption. *The Times*. Retrieved from http://www.thetimes.co.uk.

Whittle, J. (2018 July 12). Froome questions persist despite WADA's statement on handling of case. Retrieved from https://www.theguardian.com/sport/2018/jul/12/chris-froome-wada-statement-uci-handling-salbutamol-case.

Williams, R. (2016, September 23). Bradley Wiggins operated within doping rules - but rules may be wrong. *The Guardian*. Retrieved from https://www.theguardian.com/uk.

Wilson, S. (2016, September 23). Transparency is the key if clean athletes are to regain the moral high ground. *The Northern Echo*. Retrieved from http://www.thenorthernecho.co.uk/.

Ziegler, M. (2016, September 15). Froome and Wiggins medical details revealed in Russian hack. *The Times*. Retrieved from http://www.thetimes.co.uk.

Ziegler, M. (2017, March 8). Wada considers blanket ban on drug used by Wiggins. *The Times*. Retrieved from http://www.thetimes.co.uk.

Chapter 7

Substance use control at the Essendon Football Club

WADA's primary purpose is to harmonise anti-doping policy between sports and nations to ensure the equal treatment of athletes. This objective is approached using a top-down model that seeks to translate the spirit of sport into rules and regulations in the WADC by which signatories, clubs and athletes must abide. Therefore, in understanding WADA's legitimacy from a multi-level perspective, it is important to examine how doping cases can demonstrate the disconnect between macro-level policy agendas and micro-level implementation. Specifically, how failings in accountability, transparency and documentation in professional sport can cascade to create legitimacy challenges for WADA at a macro-level. The case of the Australian Sports Anti-doping Authority's (ASADA) two-year investigation into the Australian Football League (AFL) side, Essendon Football Club (EFC), and subsequent fallout provides an excellent example to explore the legitimacy dynamics between different levels of anti-doping implementation.

In 2013, ASADA investigated allegations that 34 players employed by EFC, a participant in the Australian Football League (AFL), had used banned performance-enhancing drugs (PEDs) during the 2012 season. In 2015, an independent tribunal exonerated the players and, in doing so, raised questions about WADA's ability to harmonise policy implementation between sports and nations operating under different conditions. In response, WADA appealed the decision, and in early 2016, the Court of Arbitration for Sport (CAS) judged that the club's players had used a banned substance and issued 12-month suspension notices to the players. The incident created enormous internal instability at EFC, damaged the club's reputation and traumatised the players. It also highlighted the challenges and ambiguities accompanying the task that WADA faces of creating a global anti-doping policy that is sufficiently broad to account for stakeholders with different resource and expertise levels, whilst being specific enough to account for contextual nuances. This chapter explores the EFC case and raises a series of concerns about how the decisions made by players, clubs and governing bodies can impact the legitimacy of WADA.

The EFC case reveals a complex web of contradictory claims where roles and responsibilities were confused, information flows were blocked and managerial authority was undermined. The case demonstrates that the crisis was the result of a moral failing associated with blatant cheating, while also being a consequence of management ineptitude and improper governance. Furthermore, the EFC case exemplifies the practical issues that professional sport organisations face in trying to balance the competing tensions of (1) compliance with the WADC, (2) the internal expectation of delivering high-performance and (3) protecting the brand of the league. In providing a critical analysis of the EFC case, this chapter exposes many of the ambiguities and subjectivities to which micro-level athletes and sport organisations are exposed when dealing with macro-level drug control policies and processes determined by WADA.

Anti-doping in the Australian Football League

The AFL is Australia's premier professional team sport league and is responsible for the national development of the game (AFL, 2015a). The AFL advocates for doping controls, and was one of the first professional leagues in the world to develop an anti-doping code (Horvath, 2006). The AFL's anti-doping programme was formulated within the context of the WADC, and its operational guidelines remain consistent with ASADA policy. However, this apparently seamless intersection of the WADA-ASADA-AFL relationship unravelled in early 2013 when the Australian Crime Commission (ACC) reported that questionable substance use practices and the infiltration of 'organized criminal identities' were threatening the integrity of professional sport in Australia (ACC, 2013, p. 7).

The ACC's concerns coincided with an internal review of the EFC's player supplement programme. In early 2013, EFC contacted both the AFL Commission (the sport's governing body) and ASADA to seek clarification over the legal status of its supplement programme. These liaisons materialised as a collaborative investigation into EFC by ASADA and the AFL Commission over the 2013–2015 period. EFC initiated an unsuccessful challenge into the legality of the investigation while ASADA recorded thousands of pages of evidence. In March 2015 an AFL tribunal scrutinised the evidence provided by ASADA and judged that it could not sustain the claim that the EFC player supplements programme involved the use of banned substances (AFL, 2015b). However, the matter did not end there. In response, WADA appealed the decision and sought adjudication from the CAS. In January 2016, the CAS judged that EFC players had used a banned substance and issued 12-month suspension notices (CAS, 2016). In the meantime, the reputations of senior EFC officials were destroyed, the club's governance and management systems were questioned, the integrity and good standing of the AFL was undermined, the investigative capability of ASADA was damaged and the overarching legitimacy of WADA was challenged.

The EFC drug use allegations were unique. Normally a doping violation involves a single player, but in this case an entire team of players and support staff were investigated. Yet, no positive tests were found, there was confusion over exactly what 'supplements' were being used, and there was uncertainty over whether or not the substances employed were banned during their time of use. Furthermore, the longer the EFC incident was played out, the more it 'looked like a Renaissance melodrama, inflated with bombast, caricature, shock and derision, and outraged scandal' (Carroll, 2015, p. 1).

The EFC substance use case raises a number of important governance and regulatory issues important to the legitimacy of WADA, some of which are external to EFC, and others that are embedded in the club's structure, culture and management operations. In addressing these issues, this chapter illuminates how easily doping allegations can subject WADA to the kind of scrutiny that undermines its legitimacy. Through our analysis we discuss how the EFC case can be used to understand the vulnerability of WADA's legitimacy from a multi-level perspective. WADA is dependent upon micro-level stakeholders simultaneously operating under pressure to deliver high performance whilst conforming with the macro-level idea of the spirit of sport upon which WADA is validated. The remainder of this chapter interrogates the EFC case.

Background – the key parties

Essendon Football Club

EFC, having been founded in 1872, is a membership-based sporting club that has been a participant in the AFL since its inception in 1986. Before then it was a charter member of the Victorian Football League, the forerunner of the AFL (EFC, 2015). EFC is located in a middle-class enclave in Melbourne's northern suburbs, and in 2012 had just under 50,000 members. For that year it generated an operating profit of AUS$12 million from a total revenue of AUS$65 million and accumulated AUS$35 million of net assets, making it one of the wealthiest football clubs in Australia (EFC, 2013).

In 2012, EFC employed just over 90 staff and operated under the carriage of a highly experienced board of directors featuring commercial expertise, financial acumen and football knowledge. The board included Paul Little, the managing director of Toll Holdings, one of Australia's largest transport businesses; Daryl Jackson, an internationally renowned architect with a special interest in sport stadia design; Chris Heffernan, an ex-premiership player and corporate financial advisor; and Jo-Anne Albert, a business consultant and mentor. The board chair was David Evans, who had been a long-time senior manager with two global financial corporations, Goldman Sachs and JBWere. The managing director and chief executive officer (CEO) was Ian Robson, who had been the CEO of Sport Scotland, CEO of the Leeds (UK) Rhinos (a leading English rugby league team) and the CEO the Auckland Warriors (a member of Australia's National Rugby League competition) (EFC, 2013). In 2012, the club's management system had five divisions including a football department housing a well-resourced unit in sport science and high performance.

EFC had always been a successful club with high expectations, exemplified in its motto of doing 'all that it takes' (Sharwood, 2013). This was a particularly salient mantra since the club's on-field performances had fallen below its benchmark. At the end of the 2011 season, the coaching staff of the club concluded that while players' skills and tactical know-how were satisfactory, they were vulnerable to injury and lacked physical resilience. The question that arose was what to do about it (Drane, 2014).

Australian Football League (AFL)

The AFL is both Australia's wealthiest and most popular sports league. In 2012, it generated a revenue of AUS$425 million. In addition, its net asset base was AUS$94 million, double its 2003 net asset figure of AUS$43 million (AFL, 2013b). The AFL was not only a leader in revenue generation but also a leader in the use of sport science to build better athletes (AFL, 2015; Harcourt, Marclay & Clothier, 2014). Its member clubs became 'micro-institutes of sport' as they aimed to secure a competitive edge over their rivals (Ryan, 2013).

The AFL also used its corporate resources and technological expertise to pioneer the development of anti-doping codes. In 1990, nearly 14 years before the establishment of the WADC, the AFL introduced an anti-doping code (ADC), which became a model for other sport associations and leagues (Horvath, 2006; Stewart, Dickson & Smith, 2008). The AFL ADC included a list of banned PEDs, provided for both in-season and out-of-season testing procedures, used the facilities of ASADA once it was formed and re-structured the player tribunal system in order for it to hear breaches of the code and impose sanctions for the use of banned substances.

In 1998 the AFL strengthened its ADC by inserting a two-year suspension for players found guilty of taking synthetic testosterone and other muscle-building pharmaceuticals, high-impact stimulants and diuretics as masking agents. Players who committed a second doping offence could receive a lifetime suspension (Horvath, 2006; Stewart, 2006). The AFL thus took its drug control responsibilities seriously, and in 2012, pursued a zero-tolerance approach to any type of substance use (Horvath, 2006; Stewart, Adair & Smith, 2011). The policy position appeared to work, since in-house surveys found that less than 3% of players had used banned substances over any single year (AFL, 2013).

Australian Sports Anti-Doping Authority (ASADA)

ASADA is a national government statutory authority. Its legislated mission is to protect Australia's sporting integrity through the elimination of doping, where doping is defined as the use of banned PED. Like WADA, ASADA aims to deter doping practices in sport via education, doping control, testing and advocacy (Australian Government, 2015). Its key role is to detect breaches of a sport's anti-doping policy via its testing procedures and through field investigation initiatives. Additionally, ASADA enforces breaches of policy by sanctioning anyone who violates the rules. In keeping with the operating philosophy of WADA (WADA, 2004; WADA, 2009a; WADA, 2015b), ASADA maintains that sport is a positive cultural force. Like WADA, ASADA wants to maintain the spirit of sport, which, within the 'essence of Olympism', celebrates the 'human spirit, body, and mind' (Gleaves & Llewellyn, 2013).

Australian Crime Commission (ACC)

The ACC, a government statutory authority, is Australia's national criminal intelligence agency. The aim of the ACC is to reduce the impact of crime on Australian society and the Australian economy. It has the power to conduct special investigations and operations where conventional law enforcement methods are unable or unlikely to be effective. This includes the use of Royal Commission style 'coercive powers'. The ACC deploys its crime control role by discovering, understanding and responding to the threat of serious law breaking and organised criminal activity (ACC, 2014).

The ACC became a significant player in the EFC substance use case when it released its *Organised Crime and Drugs in Sport* report in February 2013 (ACC, 2013). Prior to the drugs-in-sport report's release, the ACC provided detailed briefings to key sporting codes whom they invited to participate in the media launch (Outram, 2015). Both ASADA and the sporting codes were reminded that the ACC investigations were not about criminal arrests, charges and prosecutions, but more about the ways in which 'serious and organised criminals' had infiltrated sport and used their connections to undertake questionable practices that might threaten sport's integrity (ACC, 2013, p. 7).

Key events timeline – actions, systems and processes

Details of the EFC substance use scandal were revealed on February 5, 2013, just 10 days prior to the commencement of the AFL's pre-season fixtures. EFC announced it had contacted both ASADA and the AFL Commission to seek clarification over the legal status of its supplement use programme (Gordon, 2013; Wilson, 2013b). Under typical circumstances, supplement programmes are nothing to be concerned about, since all clubs in the major football leagues have one. The EFC programme utilised substances that were freely available over the counter, were relatively benign from a health-risk perspective and did not contain substances banned under the WADC (Outram, 2015). The EFC supplements programme initially appeared to fit within permitted guidelines (Gleeson & Niall, 2013; Hobbs & Stensholt, 2013).

After some initial uncertainty, as it turned out, EFC players had in fact injected a PED (Harcourt et al., 2014; Murphy, 2014). The questionable substance was the anti-obesity drug, AOD-9604 or Lipotropin (Heathers, 2013; Le Grand,

2015c). Lipotropin's manufacturers claimed that the substance would reduce fat and stimulate muscle growth and had been placed on WADA's banned list sometime in 2012, but it was not clear exactly when. EFC officials claimed that the club had sought advice from the AFL and ASADA on the drug's efficacy, safety and legality, although the details of when and how this transpired remained sketchy (Sharwood, 2013).

Every media outlet made the EFC supplements programme front-page news, most of it hostile (Gordon, 2013; Wilson, 2013a). A major complication emerged two days later – on February 7, 2013 – when a press conference was convened by two members of the Federal Government, Jason Clare, the minister for justice, and Kate Lundy, the minister for sport (Gordon, 2013). They were flanked by the CEOs of Australia's leading sporting bodies, together with the general manager of the ACC. The ACC used the press conference to release its report on *Organised Crime and Drugs in Sport*, which claimed that Australian sport, especially at the professional level, had a serious drug use problem. According to the ACC the problem centred on the use of peptide hormones (ACC, 2013).

The ACC claimed that growth hormone-releasing peptides (GHRPs) were used across a broad spread of sports and had become a PED of choice among many elite athletes (Koh, 2013). As the ACC noted, most GHRPs were banned under the WADA guidelines, meaning that their use 'could constitute an anti-doping rule violation' (ACC, 2013, p. 8). The substance that came under the most intensive examination was Lipotropin, which was the substance of concern for EFC officials (Le Grand, 2015c). The ACC also noted that individuals with 'extensive criminal associations' had built 'business partnerships with major Australian sporting codes' (ACC, 2013, p. 33). The evidence they declared indicated that some coaches, sports scientists and support staff had 'orchestrated and / or condoned the use of prohibited substances and methods of administration' (ACC, 2013, p. 9).

ASADA and the AFL targeted three EFC staff for interrogation. The first was James Hird, head coach and former star player with EFC. The second was Dean Robinson, the club's high-performance manager, and the third was Stephen Dank, the club's sport science director (Hemphill, 2013; Thompson, 2013). It emerged that Robertson and Dank had asked players to sign a waiver that transferred the risk of supplement use from the club to the player (CAS, 2016; Drane, 2014; Wilson, 2013c). The waiver also acted as a consent form, which implied that players receiving the supplements programme had given their approval to participate. In addition, the supplements were not only administered by injection – an unusual requirement for supplements – but were also conducted away from the club's training facility. Third, it appeared that players were not fully informed about the supplements' chemical composition, their expected physiological impact or their WADA status (Harcourt et al., 2014; Read, 2013).

As events unfolded, conflicting statements emerged, and crucial information was either not received or forgotten (Read, 2013). EFC initially claimed that neither the chief medical officer (Dr Bruce Reid) nor the head coach (Hird) were aware that players were taking experimental substances including Lipotropin (Robinson, 2013). However, it was found that while Reid was never fully briefed by Robertson and Dank, Hird was (CAS, 2016; Le Grand, 2015a). In fact, Hird and specialist coach Simon Goodwin had used the same substances as part of their own personalised supplement regimes (Wilson, 2013a). Under the guidance of Robertson and Dank, players were involved in a multi-faceted substance use programme aimed at making them stronger, leaner and more physically resilient.

In March 2013, EFC launched its own investigation into the mysterious substance use affair (Drane, 2014; Le Grand, 2015a). The aim of this review was twofold. The first was to examine the governance processes of the board of directors and determine whether the proper checks and balances had been undertaken. The second was to scrutinise the conduct of the management team in planning and executing the supplements programme. Former Telstra CEO Ziggy Switkowski headed the review and found a 'disturbing picture of a pharmacologically experimental environment never adequately controlled ... challenged... or documented within the club' (Switkowski, 2013, p. 3). The management failings became even more evident when it was found that there was 'a lack of clarity about who, exactly, was in charge of the football department' (NCAN, 2013, 4). According to Switkowski, the supplement plan was so poorly organised that it did not deserve to be called a 'plan'. He scathingly noted that if one did actually exist, it just 'evolved' and probably 'never reached a coherent, consistent shape' (NCAN, 2013, p. 1). Despite the slack management systems, Switkowski found that unconventional supplement practices did take place. He also commented that the leaders of the programme insisted that their methods were legal and compliant with ASADA's code.

Switkowski's report pointed out that a number of management processes normally associated with good governance had failed. Excessive autonomy had been given to the high-performance and sport science units, and many questionable practices were discovered. The 'diversification into exotic supplements', the 'sharp increase in frequency of injections', the shift to treatment in alternative medicine clinics, the shady emergence of 'unfamiliar suppliers' and the marginalisation of experienced medical staff – and the chief medical officer in particular – were noted (Switkowski, 2013, pp. 3–4). Switkowski also noted that while 'compliance rules existed', normal controls during an abnormal period were insufficient to check the conduct of people who may have contravened accepted procedures (NCAN, 2013, p. 4).

Club president and board chair David Evans was unable to explain the scope of management ineptitude. He apologised for the 'institutional failings', but resolved to cooperate with the investigating authorities (ABC News, 2013). He later resigned from his leadership position, following on from the departure of Ian Robson, the club's CEO. Hird, however, did not tender his resignation, and instead waited for ASADA and the AFL to act.

In August 2013, ASADA, having completed its preliminary investiga-tions, concluded that EFC had a case to answer. According to ASADA, the EFC supplements programme had exposed players to significant risk, helped to create a culture of uninformed and unregulated use of injections, did not inform players of exactly what substances were being injected into their bodies and failed to maintain even the most basic of record-keeping systems (Drane, 2014; McNicol, 2013; Murphy, 2014). ASADA also found that EFC had failed to undertake the 'normal job placement protocols' when hiring Robertson and Dank (AFL, 2013a, p. 2). The AFL Commission considered the findings, and having concluded that EFC had brought the game into disrepute, removed all their premiership points for the season, which meant that the club no longer qualified to play in the end-of-season 'finals' com-petition. The AFL Commission fined EFC AUS$2 million, stripped it of its first- and second-round draft picks for the 2014 and 2015 seasons and finally, banned Hird from coaching for the 2014 football season (Drane, 2014; Le Grand, 2014).

EFC entered the 2014 season with a new governance and management team, while the employment contracts of Robertson and Dank were not renewed. The club secured a finals appearance, but the off-field problems worsened. In June, EFC chairman Paul Little, who replaced David Evans in mid-2013, announced that the club would challenge the legality of what was believed to be a joint investigation by ASADA and the AFL, and by proxy the legitimacy of WADA. Hird took similar action on his own behalf, claiming that ASADA did not have the powers to investigate with another organisation that was, in fact, the players' employer. However, the Federal Court dismissed these appeals, and the legality of the joint investigation was upheld (Federal Court of Australia, 2014; Pierik, 2015a).

With a favourable court judgement at its side, ASADA continued its in-vestigation with the support of the AFL, and in October 2014 issued more than 30 EFC players with 'show cause' notices. The notices included evidence to suggest that the players may have used a banned PED (Kane, 2015). ASADA also invited the accused players to respond, which would be reviewed by ASADA's Anti-Doping Rule Violation Panel (ADRVP). The players were given 14 days to respond, but no one took up the invitation to reply (Pierik, 2015b).

The ADRVP finally judged that there was sufficient evidence to mount a case against the players for using a banned substance (CAS 2016; Kane, 2015). However, the offending substance was no longer AOD-9604/Lipotropin, but instead TB-500/Thymosin Beta-4 (CAS, 2016; Pierik, 2015b). Like Lipotropin, Thymosin Beta-4 is a naturally occurring peptide with the ability to promote wound-healing and muscle growth, leading to its classification as a banned substance (Koh, 2013).

In November 2014, with ADRVP advice to proceed, ASADA instructed the AFL Commission to issue 'infraction notices'. The notices declared the presence of evidence that players had breached the AFL's anti-doping rules. Players were invited to attend an AFL Tribunal hearing where decisions would be made. The three-person Tribunal Panel, chaired by former County Court judge David Jones, conducted a number of hearings and gathered significant amounts of evidence from all the key participants in the case, including EFC officials and players, the AFL Commission, ASADA and the ACC. The Tribunal handed down its decision in March 2015, more than two years after the dramatic Canberra press conference.

The decision was unanimous (AFL, 2015b; Kane, 2015; Le Grand, 2015; Pierik, 2015a). It was resolved that ASADA, which had issued the infraction notices, did not prove to a 'comfortable satisfaction' that any of the 34 EFC players had been injected with the banned substance Thymosin Beta-4. Specifically, the Tribunal was not comfortably satisfied that (1) the substance Thymosin Beta-4 was – at the relevant time – a prohibited substance under the anti-doping code; (2) any player was administered Thymosin Beta-4; and (3) any player violated clause 11.2 of the AFL Anti-Doping Code, which pertains to the use of banned substances. Consequently, the case against the EFC players was dismissed.

Although dissatisfied with the Tribunal's findings, ASADA accepted the decision and indicated that it would not appeal, aware of the inconclusive evidence (Le Grand, 2015b). WADA, however, faced with a challenge to the legitimacy of the WADC, was not prepared to concede so readily, and in early October 2015 responded with an appeal through the CAS, apparently committed as much to the symbolic action of the fight as it was to the likelihood of a successful prosecution (CAS, 2015). WADA's response repeated that abnormal levels of Thymosin Beta-4 had been found in at least two EFC players' frozen urine samples in 2012 (CAS, 2016). New EFC CEO Xavier Campbell challenged the allegation, pointing out that WADA had delivered no documentation to substantiate its claim.

In late October 2015, and after a dismal on-field season, Hird resigned. He conceded that EFC could never escape the supplements controversy while he remained coach, and had decided to fall honourably upon his sword. An alternative interpretation of Hird's decision was that his management of the team's performance was unsatisfactory, and that any head coach in a similar predicament would have had their services terminated. Additionally, the AFL Tribunal found Dank guilty of 10 charges of misconduct, with his reputation damaged beyond repair.

In the meantime, CAS re-scheduled the WADA appeal, and in January 2016 presented its judgement. It reversed the AFL Tribunal's decision to exonerate the 34 EFC players, and suspended them for one year. The CAS judgement both shocked and confused the EFC staff and players (Hird, 2016; Niall, 2016). CAS not only used the same evidence supplied to the AFL Tribunal but also used the same principle of being 'comfortably satisfied' when making their decision (CAS, 2016; Kane, 2016).

Issues affecting legitimacy – structures and explanations

The EFC case raised issues that went beyond concerns about drug-related cheating, moral laxity and a single-minded drive to do all that it takes, whatever the consequences. A critical reading of the relevant reports and documents suggests that the catastrophe that enveloped the EFC was mainly the result of managerial failures that cumulatively destroyed the credibility and legitimacy of all the key stakeholders. These managerial failures undermined the legitimacy of WADA as they typified the performance-focused beliefs underpinning the values of elite sport in contrast to the spirit of sport used to frame the WADC. Furthermore, specific, inter-related themes can be identified within the managerial failures of the EFC case: (1) governance; (2) accountability, transparency, and communication; and (3) timeliness and due process.

Governance

While management processes shape the day-to-day performance of professional team sport organisations, their vision, strategy and culture are determined by governance systems (Naimo, 2014). Governance involves processes and practices that allow an organisation to achieve maximum value for stakeholders by setting policies and direction, exercising power, and determining how decisions are made and how resources are deployed (Hoye, Smith, Nicholson & Stewart, 2015). In the case of EFC's supplements programme, questions regularly arose as to whether sound governance practices were in place.

Both the board and the club's senior management team were highly credentialed, and it appeared that the governance and management structures were clearly defined and transparent. However, the 2013 internal review revealed the aforementioned 'disturbing picture', further accentuated by apparent management failings that became even more evident when 'a lack of clarity about who, exactly, was in charge of the football department' was exposed (Switkowski, 2013, p. 4). The review further noted that, 'a number of management processes normally associated with good governance had failed during this period' (Switkowski, 2013, p. 5). Some of these failings included concerns about how EFC was running its football operations, especially the excessive autonomy given to the high-performance and sport science units. Specifically noted was 'the diversification into exotic supplements, the sharp increase in frequency of injections, the shift to treatment offsite in alternative medicine clinics, the shady emergence of unfamiliar suppliers, and the marginalisation of traditional medical staff' (CAS, 2016; Wilson, 2013b, p. 1).

Weak governance can also create systemic problems throughout an organisation, beginning with a cavalier approach to risk management and associated legal issues (Milot, 2014). *Risk management* refers to the mitigation of accidents and injuries, and the responsible management of the settings in which sporting events and programmes take place (Cotten & Wolohan, 2009; Thorpe, Buti, Davies, Fridman & Jonson, 2013). The goal of risk management is twofold: to provide for the safety of everyone involved in an activity (including participants, spectators and officials) and to reduce or limit losses to the organisation. EFC appeared to jettison its responsibilities in these areas. As ASADA observed (ASADA, 2013; Murphy, 2014), the EFC supplements programme exposed players to significant risk, helped to create a culture of uninformed and unregulated use of injections, did not inform players of exactly what substances were being injected into their bodies and failed to maintain even the most basic of record-keeping systems. These failed responsibilities extended into staff management, since EFC had not undertaken appropriate recruitment protocols when hiring two influential but controversial sport scientists (CAS, 2016).

Further complications arose when Dank asked players to sign a waiver that transferred the 'risk of use' from the club to the player (Stewart, 2013). The waiver was designed as an informed consent declaration, the implication being that players were afforded the opportunity to evaluate the new supplements programme and then to consent or not, in the absence of any coercion pressures. In reality, players were not fully informed about the nature of the supplements, their chemical compositions and physical effects and where they fell within WADA regulations (Le Grand, 2015a; McNicol, 2013). In light of the conflicting information about how the process transpired, it was unlikely that the consent secured was in fact informed (Le Grand, 2015a).

A likely absence of informed consent also raises the probability of negligence from the club, and in particular, the sport scientists. Negligence is an unintentional tort that injures a person, property or reputation caused by a failure to use the level of care a reasonably prudent person would use under similar circumstances. In this case, players had allegedly been given a 'mysterious cocktail of supplements during the 2012 season' (Stewart, 2013, p. 1), some of which were untested and had not been properly trialled. This raised many concerns. Firstly, did the substances deliver what they claimed to? Secondly, were the supplements safe from side effects that might have undermined the health of the players? Finally, could the products be used, being approved under the AFL's anti-doping rules?

The governance practices implemented (or not) by EFC in the pursuit of success are far removed from the sporting ideals stipulated in the WADC and exemplify the vulnerability of WADA's legitimacy to challenge from micro-level implementation. From a multi-level legitimacy perspective, strong legitimacy is derived from a high level of consensus between stakeholders about the appropriateness of an organisation or behaviour. In this case, the macro-level spirit of sport approach to anti-doping propagated by WADA and supported by the IOC and select governments is at odds with the reality faced by elite sport organisations.

Accountability, transparency and communication

In examining this case, it was never clear as to who was accountable for the entire scenario, who approved the supplements programme, who organised its implementation or who monitored its operation. Blame was shifted with every revelation and exposé (Gottliebsen, 2013; Le Grand, 2015a).

The organisational structure of EFC met the principles of conventional design. The club's hierarchy positioned players at the base and linked them to a defined school of supervisors encompassing coaches, sport scientists, medical personnel and high-performance staff, who were responsible for player progress and productivity. These supervisors reported to middle management, which, in this case, included the football department manager, staff operations manager and the senior coach. Middle management, in turn, served as the conduit to their CEO, who reported to the board of directors, who had ultimate responsibility for the strategic intent of the club. Yet, it was never clear who exactly was accountable for the operation of the supplements programme. ASADA argued that the players should have been accountable for knowing what was going into their bodies, even if their supervisors advised that the supplements were safe and permissible. While EFC officials argued that players had given their consent, the AFL Tribunal found that the coaches and sport scientists had not always acted on their moral and legal obligation to ensure the health and safety of players (Sharwood, 2013).

WADA responded to the accountability problem when updating its code in 2014, declaring that supervisory personnel and support staff should have greater accountability for supplement use (Harcourt et al., 2014). WADA argued that sport managers should be made accountable for governance failures that increase the risk of doping (Harcourt et al., 2014). However, evidently these accountability principles were never adopted by EFC (CAS, 2016).

A major part of the communication breakdown was also linked to improper record-keeping, especially in the area of programme monitoring (Switkowski, 2013). There were no records of the substances or dosages injected, the number of injections, when injections were given or any illnesses or negative reactions from the substances (Le Grand, 2015a). Without appropriate record-keeping, it is impossible to locate the ethical and operational balance between managing players' health and their performance (Dijkstra, Pollock, Chakraverty & Alonso, 2014). As such, EFC failed to integrate the performance, health management and coaching programmes, and was thus susceptible to synergy depletion, under-achievement, a loss of focus and a major organisational breakdown (Dijkstra, et al., 2014). EFC failed to maintain even the most basic of record-keeping systems, and consequently had no rational process for monitoring the player supplement programme and measuring its performance. The risk presented to athletes subject to the poorly monitored supplements programme and WADA's reliance on the ability of clubs to effectively organise a safe supplements system highlights the discord between the WADC policy and the challenges faced by those responsible for implementation.

Timeliness and due process

Beyond the failures already identified, there are also questions about the time-liness of the ASADA investigation and the extent to which due process was followed prior to the AFL Tribunal decision (Gottliebsen, 2013). It took three years to bring the case to resolution, which resulted from an appeal by WADA and a judgement by CAS that reversed the AFL Tribunal decision to exonerate the players. Due process is a course of legal proceedings according to rules and principles established by jurisprudence for the protection and enforcement of private rights (Cotten & Wolohan, 2009). A first relevant form is substantive due process, where rules and regulations should be fair and reasonable and protect individuals from arbitrary and capricious actions (Cotten & Wolohan, 2009). A second is procedural due process, where the methods used to enforce the rules and regulations and determine violations and sanctions will ensure fair treatment for every individual (Cotten & Wolohan, 2009). While substantive due process was followed, there were claims that procedural due process had not been followed by ASADA in its attempt to maximise the evidence base from which to launch a prosecution (Hird, 2016).

The gap between policy and practice

This case highlights the complexities involved for WADA in handling in-cidents of this nature. No shortage of views was aired as to why the EFC case became so complicated, and there was continual disagreement on what really went on in the dealings between the AFL Commission and ASADA. There was surprise over how the CAS judgement could so easily override the AFL Tribunal decision, while the arguments raged as to who was ultimately responsible for the whole fiasco. The only consensus was that the legitimacy of each organisation was undermined.

Notwithstanding these complications between policy and practice, the EFC substance use case has significant implications for the management of doping incidents and the legitimacy of WADA. First, problems will inevitably arise when supplements are used without proper knowledge about their contents, efficacy and credibility. There is a litany of incidents involving the inadvertent use of banned substances through supplement use, and subsequent player sus-pensions for doping (Outram & Stewart, 2015). Under WADA regulations, the gap that inadvertent use of PED via contaminated supplements fell into is closed, and it is now understood that 'player pleading' about the fact that a banned substance was not listed on the packet or container is no defence, and the suspension will stand (CAS, 2016; WADA, 2009b; WADA, 2015a, 2015b). However, in this case, the new policy was too little too late.

Second, players have the right to know what they are ingesting, and super-visors who fail to provide informed consent are derelict in their professional responsibilities (Le Grand 2015a, 2015c; Stewart & Smith, 2014). In the EFC case, players were ill-informed on technical issues, and were therefore vulnerable to the pronouncements of sport scientists, medical officers, coaches, trainers and peers (Hemphill, 2013). A pivotal argument for anti-doping and the prohibition of select substances is the protection of an athlete's health. Therefore, the risk presented to players who were not adequately informed posed a threat to WADA's ability to protect athletes.

Third, ongoing intra-organisational collaboration is crucially important when dealing with substance use if WADA and other stakeholders' legitimacy is to be safeguarded from unnecessary challenge arising from poor policy compliance. In this case, EFC's communication network was distorted beyond coherence and as a result, the substance injection programme was not fully understood by almost everybody who had an interest in the matter (Hobbs & Stensholt, 2013; Le Grand, 2015c; Switkowski, 2013a). Moreover, sport scientists – the players' supervisors – had excessive autonomy and were free to engineer their own player improvement programmes. In addition, the board of directors, coaching panel and medical staff failed to ensure that WADA rules were not broken, or that player rights were not abused. The potential abuse of player rights under organisations subject to the WADC again undermines WADA's legitimacy. Fourth, the enormous media coverage that surrounded the EFC case – with most of it being highly critical – highlights the importance of proactive crisis management; when the media sets the communication agenda, the risk of reputational harm is high. Unsubstantiated rumours and ideologically driven commentary not only shaped the public response but also reduced complex substance use policy analysis to simplistic arguments and inflammatory moral judgements (Le Grand, 2015a). The simplification of nuanced anti-doping issues to simplistic moral judgements poses a threat to WADA's perceived legitimacy if it were to influence public support and attitudes towards anti-doping.

Fifth, a lack of openness and failure to acknowledge responsibility for the problem can often only widen the reputational damage. Not only were EFC players, coaches, managers and the board of directors damaged, but every stakeholder also had their goodwill shaken and reputations tarnished (Hird, 2016; Niall, 2016). The actions of the AFL Commission and ASADA, and especially the regular leaking of confidential information, also called into question the integrity of their processes (Le Grand, 2015a). A complex causal web involving the moral laxity of EFC officials, the club's management failings, ASADA's relentless drive to secure a win and WADA's single-minded response to enacting punishment all conspired to undermine the moral legitimacy of these organisations to manage anti-doping regulations and procedures.

Conclusion

It is evident throughout the exploration of the EFC case that there was a disconnect between the ideals of anti-doping stated in the WADC and the organisational environment at EFC. There is no single explanation for the

EFC's massive mismanagement of its supplements programme. Multiple causes, both contextual and internal to the club's management systems, fuelled the crisis and destroyed the club's operational effectiveness. These factors were encapsulated in the conduct of Robertson and Dank, who brought to the club a hyper-competitive ethos that prioritised on-field success over administrative procedures, secret deals over symmetrical information flows and quick perfor- mance fixes over the protection of player welfare (CAS, 2016; Hird, 2016). As a result, formal reporting arrangements, transparent information flows and con- sultative decision-making processes were sacrificed at the altar of doing all it takes to secure a competitive edge (Carroll, 2015; Switkowski, 2013). Internally, a climate that legitimised 'doing all that it takes' (EFC, 2012) was doomed to fail. Not only were players treated as human machines (Lopez, 2012), but the language of science and technology was also used to camouflage knowledge and evidence gaps (Le Grand, 2015a; Waddington, 2015). In doing so, a gap emerged between the prescribed ideals of sport and the reality of elite, commercial sport business.

As a primer for effective sport anti-doping governance under WADA in the future, the core message is to not be side-tracked by seeking simple solutions to complex problems, but instead see opportunities for legitimacy and success through the strategic and operational prisms of accountability, transparency and documentation. WADA faces the challenge of creating a global anti-doping policy that accounts for inter-stakeholder differences in resource and expertise levels, whilst being specific enough to harmonise implementation between signatories. This case reveals that doping is a complex problem involving multiple actors and operational factors that are not necessarily suited to a one-size-fits-all policy. In future, WADA may need to re-evaluate the balance it strikes between specificity and flexibility to safeguard its legitimacy. The per- ipheral message is to be acutely aware of the ways in which inept management can expose organisations such as EFC, ASADA and WADA to serious harm, and understand how proper risk-management, good governance and strong systems of transparency and accountability can be used as a bulwark against the corrupting influence of unprincipled hyper-competition.

References

ABC News (2013, May 7). Bombers apologise for 'institutional failings'. Retrieved from http://www.abc.net.au/news/2013-05-06/essendon-releases-report-findings/4671934.
Australian Crime Commission (ACC). (2013). *Organised crime and drugs in sport: New generation performance and image enhancing drugs and organised criminal involvement in their use in professional sports.* Canberra: Australian Crime Commission. Retrieved from https://www.crimecommission.gov.au/sites/default/files/organised-crime-and-drugs-in-sports-feb2013.pdf.
Australian Crime Commission. (2014). *Annual Report: 2013-2014.* Canberra: ACC. Retrieved from https://www.crimecommission.gov.au/annual-report-2013-2014.

Australian Football League (AFL). (2013a). *Essendon Football Club – Notice of charge.* Melbourne: AFL. Retrieved from http://www.afl.com.au/staticfile/AFL%20Tenant/AFL/Files/EssendonFC-notice-of-charges.pdf.

Australian Football League (AFL). (2013b). *Annual report 2012.* Melbourne: AFL. Retrieved from http://www.afl.com.au/staticfile/AFL%20Tenant/AFL/Files/AFL%20 Annual%20Report%202012_web.pdf.

Australian Football League (AFL). (2015a). The AFL explained: Past and present. Retrieved from http://www.afl.com.au/afl-hq/the-afl-explained.

Australian Football League (AFL). (2015b, March 31). Full statement from the AFL's Anti-Doping Tribunal. Retrieved from http://www.afl.com.au/news/2015-03-31/full-tribunal-statement.

Australian Government. About Australian Sports Anti-doping Authority - ASADA. Retrieved December 23, 2015, from https://www.asada.gov.au/about-asada.

Australian Sports Anti-Doping Authority (ASADA). (2013). *Annual report for 2012.* Canberra: ASADA.

Carroll, J. (2015, December 26) Essendon drugs saga: Renaissance melodrama fouls the air. *Weekend Australian,* pp. 34–35. Retrieved from http://www.theaustralian.com.au/news/inquirer/essendon-drugs-saga-renaissance-melodrama-fouls-the-air/news-story/6d6c7fdb2928f0f51cf86a55470e2bc3.

Cotten, D.J. & Wolohan, J. (2009). *Law for recreation and sport managers* (3rd ed.). Dubuque, IA: Kendall-Hunt.

CAS. (2015). *The Court of Arbitration for Sport (CAS) to issue its decision in the Essendon Case in January 2016.* Retrieved from http://www.tas-cas.org/fileadmin/user_upload/Media_Release_4059_221215.pdf.

CAS. (2016). *World Anti-Doping Agency v. Thomas Bellchambers et al., Australian Football League, Australian Sports anti-Doping Authority: Arbitral award delivered by the Court of Arbitration for Sport.* Retrieved from http://www.tas-cas.org/fileadmin/user_upload/Arbitral_Award_WADA_ESSENDON.pdf.

Dijkstra, H.P., Pollock, N., Chakraverty, R. & Alonso, J.M. (2014). Managing the health of the elite athlete: A new integrated performance health management and coaching model. *British Journal of Sports Medicine, 48*(7), 523–531.

Drane, R. (2014, May 14). Whatever they took. *Inside Sport,* 43–50.

EFC. (2013). *Annual report 2013.* Melbourne: EFC.

EFC. (2015). *History.* Retrieved from http://www.essendonfc.com.au/club/history

Federal Court of Australia. (2014, August 4) *Essendon Football Club v Chief Executive Officer of the Australian Sports Anti-Doping Authority [2014] FCA 1019.* Retrieved from http://www.fedcourt.gov.au/_.

Gleaves, J. & Llewellyn, M. (2013). Sport, drugs and amateurism: Tracing the real cultural origins of anti-doping rules in international sport. *The International Journal of the History of Sport, 31*(8), 839–853.

Gleeson, M. & Niall, J. (2013, February 6). Essendon engulfed by drug controversy. *The Age,* p. 2. Retrieved from http://www.theage.com.au/afl/afl-news/essendon-engulfed-by-drug-controversy-20130205-2dwmb.html.

Gordon, M. (2013, February 8). This is the blackest day in Australian sport. *The Age.* Retrieved from http://www.smh.com.au/national/this-is-the-blackest-day-in-australian-sport-20130207-2e1i3.html.

Gottliebsen, R. (2013, July 17). Sports drugs debacle falls on ASADA shoulders. *Business Spectator*, Retrieved from http://www.businessspectator.com.au/print/540661.

Harcourt, P.R., Marclay, F. & Clothier, B. (2014). A forensic perspective of the AFL investigation into peptides: An anti-doping investigation case study. *British Journal of Sports Medicine*, 8(10), 810–813.

Heathers, J. (2013, February 8). Essendon faces a doping investigation … but what are peptides? *The Conversation*. Retrieved from http://theconversation.com/essendon-faces-a-doping-investigation-but-what-are-peptides-12042.

Hemphill, D. (2013, February 12). Doping shock: Pointing the finger at sport scientists. *The Conversation*. Retrieved from http://theconversation.com/doping-shock-pointing-the-finger-at-sports-scientists-12129.

Hird, J. (2016, January 15). We were duped. *Herald Sun*, 6.

Hobbs, M. & Stensholt, J. (2013, February 9–10). Directors fear breach over drugs claims. *The Australian Financial Review: Weekend Edition*, p. 1. Retrieved from http://www.afr.com/business/directors-fear-breach-over-drugs-claims-20130209-je923.

Horvath, P. (2006) Anti-doping and human rights in sport: The case of the AFL and the WADA Code. *Monash University Law Review*, 32(2), 358–359.

Hoye, R., Smith, A., Nicholson, M. & Stewart, B. (2015). *Sport management: Principles and applications* (4th ed.). London: Routledge.

Kane, D. (2015, April 24) Why ASADA's case against Essendon players fell apart. *The Age*, p. 1. Retrieved from http://www.theage.com.au/afl/afl-news/why-asadas-case-against-essendon-players-fell-apart-20150424-1mrc4l.html.

Kane, D. (2016, January 16). The mystery of the CAS verdict. *The Age*, p. 47.

Koh, B. (2013, March 7). Cronulla Sharks and thymosin beta-4 … is it doping? *The Conversation*. Retrieved from http://theconversation.com/cronulla-sharks-and-thymosin-beta-4-is-it-doping-12694.

Le Grand, C. (2014, June 3). After 16 months, we still don't know if Essendon Bombers used banned drugs. *The Australian*. Retrieved from http://www.theaustralian.com.au/sport/afl/after-16-months-we-still-dont-know-if-essendon-bombers-used-banned-drugs/story-fnca0u4y-1226940801757.

Le Grand, C. (2015a). *The straight dope book: The inside story of sport's biggest drug scandal*. Melbourne: Melbourne University Press.

Le Grand, C. (2015b, June 3–4). ASADA's flimsy case was always dead in the water. *The Weekend Australian*, p. 12.

Le Grand, C. (2015c, April 4–5). No evidence for Jobe Admission. *The Weekend Australian*, p. 33.

Lopez, B. (2012). Doping as technology: A rereading of the history of performance-enhancing substance use in the light of Brian Winston's interpretative model for technological continuity and change. *International Journal of Sport Policy and Politics*, 4(1), 55–71.

McNicol, A. (2013). *Essendon charges revealed*. AFL. Retrieved December 23, 2015, from http://www.afl.com.au/news/2013-08-21/afl-reveals-charges.

Milot, L. (2014). Ignorance, harm, and the regulation of performance enhancing substances. *Journal of Sports and Entertainment Law*, 15, 92–146.

Murphy, J. (2014, November 13). Federal Court upholds the legality of the 'joint' AFL–ASADA investigation into Essendon. *FlagPost: Commonwealth Parliamentary Library*. Retrieved from http://parlinfo.aph.gov.au/parlInfo/download/library/prspub/3536643/

upload_binary/3536643.pdf;fileType=application%2Fpdf#search=%22library/prspub/
3536643%22.

Naimo, J. (2014). Ethics and the art of sport governance. Achieving ethical excellence. *Research in Ethical Issues in Organizations, 12*, 91–112.

News Corp Australia Network (NCAN) (2013, May 6). Full text of the publicly released Ziggy Switkowski report after his review of governance at Essendon FC. *Herald Sun*. Retrieved from http://www.heraldsun.com.au/sport/afl/full-text-of-the-publicly-released-ziggy-switkowski-report-after-his-review-of-governance-at-essendon-fc/story-e6frf9l6-1226635955142.

Niall, J. (2016, January 13) Game over. *The Age*, p. 2.

Outram, S.M. (2015). Protecting sport from itself: a critical analysis of the 2013 Australian Crime Commission's Report into crime and drugs in sport. *International Journal of Sport Policy and Politics, 7*(4), 605–622.

Outram, S.M. & Stewart, B. (2015). Doping through supplement use: A review of the available empirical data. *International Journal of Sport Nutrition and Exercise Metabolism, 25*(1), 54–59.

Pierik. J. (2015a, March 31). Essendon supplements saga: Your guide to Tuesday's AFL anti-doping verdict. *The Age*. Retrieved from http://www.theage.com.au/afl/afl-news/essendon-supplements-saga-your-guide-to-tuesdays-afl-antidoping-verdict-20150330-1majjd.html.

Pierik. J. (2015b). Thymosin beta 4 not on WADA banned list: Stephen Dank. *The Age*. 29 March. Retrieved from http://www.theage.com.au/afl/afl-news/thymosin-beta-4-not-on-wada-banned-list-stephen-dank-20150329-1ma7do.html.

Read, B. 2013. Show us the drug abuse evidence. *Weekend Australian*, 9 February, p. 35.

Robinson, M. (2013) Reid all about it. *Herald Sun*, 27 June. Retrieved from http://www.heraldsun.com.au/sport/afl/why-essendon-coach-james-hird-is-backing-club-doctor-dr-bruce-reid/story-fni5f6kv-1226670436793.

Ryan, P. (2013) *Inside the world of sport science*. Retrieved from http://www.afl.com.au/news/2013-03-15/inside-the-world-of-afl-sport-science.

Sharwood, A. (2013, February 5). Bombshell: The slogan that's too close to home. *Herald Sun*, pp. 2–4. Retrieved from http://www.heraldsun.com.au/sport/afl/bombshell-the-slogan-thats-too-close-to-home/story-e6frf9l6-1226570963213.

Stewart, B. (2013, February 10). Essendon scandal a symptom of Australia's sporting woes. *The Conversation*. Retrieved from http://theconversation.com/essendon-scandal-a-symptom-of-australias-sporting-woes-12085.

Stewart, B., Adair, D. & Smith, A. (2011). Drivers of illicit drug use in Australian sport, *Sport Management Review, 14*(1), 1–10.

Stewart, B. & Smith, A. (2014). *Rethinking drug use in sport: Why the war on drugs in sport will never be won*. London: Routledge.

Stewart, R. (2006). The World Anti-Doping Agency and the AFL. In M. Nicholson, R. Hess & R. Stewart (Eds.), *Football fever: Moving the goalposts* (pp. 107–114). Hawthorne, Australia: Maribyrnong Press.

Stewart, R., Dickson, G. & Smith, A. (2008). Drug use in the Australian Football League: A critical survey. *Sporting Traditions: The Journal of the Australian Society for Sports History, 25*(2), 50–66.

Switkowski, Z. (2013). *Dr. Ziggy Switkowski report. Essendon Football Club – Review findings and recommendations.* Retrieved December 23, 2015, from http://www.essendonfc.com.au/news/2013-05-06/dr-ziggy-switkowski-report.

Thompson, K. (2013, February 13). Sports science: Time for proper accreditation. *The Conversation.* Retrieved from http://theconversation.com/sports-science-time-for-proper-accreditation-12095.

Thorpe, D., Buti, A., Davies, C., Fridman, S., & Jonson, P.F. (2013). *Sports law* (2nd ed.). Oxford: Oxford University Press.

WADA. (2004). Strategic plan 04-09. *World Anti-Doping Agency.* Retrieved from https://www.wada-ama.org/en/.

WADA. (2009a). Strategic plan 09-14. *World Anti-Doping Agency.* Retrieved from https://www.wada-ama.org/en/.

WADA. (2009b). Anti-doping code. *World Anti-Doping Agency.* Retrieved from https://www.wada-ama.org/en/.

WADA. (2015a.) Anti-doping code. *World Anti-Doping Agency.* Retrieved from https://www.wada-ama.org/en/.

WADA. (2015b). Who we are? *World Anti-Doping Agency.* Retrieved from https://www.wada-ama.org/en/who-we-are.

Waddington, I. (2015). Towards an understanding of drug use in sport: A medical sociological perspective. In V. Moller, I. Waddington, & J. Hoberman (Eds.), *Routledge handbook of drugs and sport* (pp. 405–418). London: Routledge.

Wilson, C. (2013a, March 16). Dons did not check Dank. *The Age.* Retrieved from http://www.theage.com.au/afl/afl-news/dons-did-not-check-dank-20130315-2g69u.html.

Wilson, C. (2013b, February 11). Nine clubs vulnerable on drugs. *The Age,* pp. 1–2.

Wilson, C. (2013c, February 9). Australian doping authorities have dropped the ball. *Saturday Age,* p. 2 [Sports].

Chapter 8

Recreational drugs

As we continue to examine issues and policies that have challenged WADA's legitimacy as the regulator of anti-doping, this chapter will focus on how the prohibition of recreational drugs has led to debate about its appropriate jurisdiction. *Recreational drugs*, also termed *social drugs*, *illicit substances* or *substances of abuse*, are distinguished from PEDs because although they may offer ergogenic benefits in certain circumstances, they are most commonly used for non-performance-enhancing reasons (e.g., in social situations). Problematically, the alternative terms listed here reflect biased assumptions about the nature and use of recreational drugs. Substances of abuse can be viewed as stigmatising and implies addiction, social drugs limit the full spectrum of use excluding other motives (e.g., medicinal purposes) and illicit substances do not provide sufficient differentiation from PEDs. In response, we use the term *recreational drugs* in this chapter because it denotes a substance that might be taken for a variety of reasons, but not typically for performance enhancement. As we will demonstrate, WADA's decision to adopt a punitive, prohibitive approach to recreational drugs has been a source of criticism and challenge and demonstrates the organisation's narrow policy approach.

Recreational drug classes prohibited by WADA include cannabinoids such as marijuana, narcotics such as methadone and stimulants such as cocaine. Prohibition of recreational drugs has long presented a significant challenge to the legitimacy of WADA, because these substances do not reflect doping in the typical sense of cheating to gain an advantage (Waddington, Christiansen, Gleaves, Hoberman & Møller, 2013). Originally classified and prohibited in the same manner as other PED groups, such as anabolic agents (e.g., stanozolol the drug Ben Johnson tested positive for in 1988), little evidence suggests that recreational substances deliver performance-enhancing benefits (Heuberger & Cohen, 2019). The caveat that WADA has made for recreational drugs is that they are only prohibited 'in-competition'. In the 2015 WADC, for an infringement to occur in-competition, an athlete needs to submit a doping control sample in a 12-hour period prior to an event in which they are participating through to the end of any sample collection process for the competition. From the 2021 WADC, the start point for in-competition testing will be considered as

11:59 p.m. on the day before competition begins. An out-of-competition (OOC) test encompasses any other time. The rationale for the in-competition ban is that the effects of cannabinoids, stimulants and narcotics may offer temporary or indirect performance benefits such as reducing pain or pre-competition anxiety. Despite the absence of evidence for ergogenic effects, athletes could still face up to a two-year ban after testing positive for the presence of a recreational substance in a sample provided in-competition, even if the substance was used OOC. As Waddington and Møller (2019) noted, WADA's decision to place punishments on the use of recreational drugs has

> redefined what constitutes 'doping' in a way which means that, for the first time, athletes can be punished for a form of behaviour – the use of a recreational drug which is not performance-enhancing – which almost nobody would regard as cheating and which does not constitute 'doping' in any meaningful sense of the term.
>
> (p. 222)

The perceived injustice of sanctioning athletes after testing positive for recreational drugs that were neither taken for performance-enhancing reasons nor conferred any in-competition benefit has led to regular critiques of the policy (e.g., International Network of Humanistic Doping Research, 2013). WADA's position also contrasts the increasingly liberal attitudes towards recreational drug regulation in Western society (Felson, Adamczyk & Thomas, 2019), indicated by the growing cadre of regions and countries like Canada and Portugal that have legalised possession of substances such as cannabis.

The 2021 version of the WADC reflects changing attitudes towards recreational drugs policy. For the first time, athletes who can prove that they took a recreational drug OOC for reasons unrelated to performance will receive a three-month ban (WADC, 2020). The reduction in the period of ineligibility reflects a permissive shift in WADA's attitude towards recreational drug use following the legitimacy challenges prohibition has generated. As this chapter will discuss, the penalty reduction nevertheless exemplifies WADA's limited scope for change. We demonstrate that WADA's response to the legitimacy challenge created by recreational drugs fails to move beyond the policy choices constrained by its philosophical roots in the spirit of sport and Olympism, as seen in the recent revisions to the WADC.

To analyse the relationship between WADA's legitimacy and recreational drug prohibition, the remainder of this chapter is structured as follows. Firstly, the reasons for recreational drug prohibition are discussed, accompanied by critiques of prohibition and estimates of recreational drug use in athlete populations. Secondly, a case study is presented of Peruvian footballer and national team captain Paolo Guerrero. Guerrero's case is illustrative of the complexity of recreational drug regulation and the legitimacy challenges prohibition raises for WADA. In 2017, Guerrero tested positive for the cocaine metabolite (a molecule produced in a biological chemical reaction) benzoylecgonine, said to be unintentionally ingested by drinking tea. Guerrero received a six-month ban from FIFA, later extended to 14 months by the Court of Arbitration for Sport (CAS) following an appeal by WADA. Guerrero was set to miss captaining Peru in the 2018 FIFA World Cup Finals tournament, Peru's first finals appearance since 1982. It was only through the public support of other participating teams and interjection by the Swiss Federal Tribunal to temporarily suspend Guerrero's period of ineligibility that he was able to participate. Finally, the chapter will discuss WADA's most recent changes to the WADC, what the revisions illustrate about how the organisation can respond to legitimacy challenges and the impact this has on athletes. The discussion concludes that WADA operates with limited scope to accommodate alternative approaches that may better protect athletes.

Justifying prohibition

Like all other substances that are prohibited by WADA, recreational drugs are banned with reference to three criteria. Firstly, is the substance performance enhancing? Secondly, is the substance detrimental to an athlete's health? Thirdly, does use of the substance violate the spirit of sport? If any two of these criteria are met, a substance or method can be prohibited. The first two questions are difficult to answer as rigorous, high-quality scientific evidence is required to determine a reliable verdict. Yet it is the third question that has primarily drawn criticism for determining the legality of a substance, as it relies on social and ethical judgements. The *spirit of sport* has become a term representing the characteristics and values of the Olympics, which the WADC states as:

> Health; Ethics, fair play and honesty; Athletes' rights as set forth in the Code; Excellence in performance; Character and Education; Fun and joy; Teamwork; Dedication and commitment; Respect for rules and laws; Respect for self and other Participants; Courage; and Community and solidarity.
>
> (WADC, 2020, p. 13)

According to WADA, all the values listed constitute the spirit of sport, and therefore, any substance that could jeopardise these values risks prohibition. Arguments supporting the prohibition of recreational drugs in-competition have been based on variations of the three assessment criteria.

The potential negative health effects of recreational drug misuse on athletes and the general population have been the primary argument used to justify prohibition and the associated punishments for transgressions. Reviewing clinical evidence, long-term misuse of recreational substances, such as cannabinoids, may lead to long-term social and physical harm (Crean, Crane &

Mason, 2011). Furthermore, it has been claimed that athletes function as community role models, and that their use of recreational substances might encourage children and adolescents to duplicate the behaviour. A clear example of this attitude is offered by the three-month ban given to US swimmer and most successful Olympian ever Michael Phelps. In 2009 USA Swimming suspended Phelps after a picture emerged of him with a marijuana pipe at a party. Despite not committing an anti-doping rule violation, USA Swimming justified his suspension because Phelps was considered a prominent role model: 'We decided to send a strong message to Michael because he disappointed so many people, particularly the hundreds of thousands of USA Swimming member kids who look up to him as a role model and hero' (Macur, 2009). In addition to USA Swimming not providing financial support to Phelps for three months, cereal brand Kellogg's decided not to renew its sponsorship deal with Phelps following the incident. From a role model perspective, the prohibition of recreational drugs provides a wider societal benefit regardless of performance enhancement (Henne, Koh & McDermott, 2013; Lentillon-Kaestner, 2013).

In terms of performance enhancement, the ergogenic benefits of recreational drugs have been argued to encompass psychological boosts as well as physiological adaptation, including before, during and after training and/or competition. Therefore, the psychological effects of recreational drugs such as increased concentration, pain relief and mood alteration constitute performance enhancement (Lentillon-Kaestner, 2013). For instance, an athlete who uses cannabis to manage pain from training and relax from the pressures of competition might be said to receive an unfair performance advantage.

Finally, the spirit of sport has been claimed as a critical assessment criterion on the grounds that without it doping would no longer be treated as unethical behaviour, but rather a medical behaviour determined by harm criteria (McNamee, 2012). If this were the case, adequately defining 'harm' would be just as problematic as defining the spirit of sport because harm and health can be conceptualised in many forms and from multiple ethical perspectives (McNamee, 2012). The spirit of sport as a criterion has also been defended because it enables approval, as well as prohibition, of substances and methods that may otherwise be banned on narrower criteria advocated by some critics. For example, should a substance or method that offers performance enhancement, is safe to use, but requires no active effort from the athlete to gain any benefit still be prohibited? With the inclusion of the spirit of sport, it is possible to prohibit this substance under two out of the three criteria. It would not be possible if performance enhancement and harm to the athlete were the only criteria.

The argument for the specific prohibition of cannabis provided by Huestis, Mazzoni and Rabin (2011) (the last two authors being WADA employees at the time of the article's publication) is informative about the logic underpinning prohibition. Huestis et al. (2011) pointed out that based on the available data of 'the effects of acute and chronic cannabis exposure, cannabis fulfils the criterion of potential for health risks' (p. 954), and that 'cannabis can be performance enhancing for some athletes and sports disciplines' (p. 956). Considering the more subjective appraisal of whether cannabis use violates the spirit of sport, cannabis' illegal status in some countries and the expectation that athletes should function as role models are deemed sufficient to satisfy the spirit of sport criteria. For these reasons, cannabis is banned in-competition. Likewise, Bergamaschi and Crippa (2013) supported the same line of reasoning, proposing further restrictions on recreational drugs in order to protect athletes from harm. The problem with the in-competition ban on cannabinoids lies in determining exactly when an athlete uses a substance, and whether it is on the day of competition (Saugy et al., 2006).

Given that the arguments for recreational drug prohibition predominantly rely upon a line of reasoning linked to athlete and societal welfare, it is instructive to examine the prevalence of recreational drug use in athlete populations to assess the scale of the alleged problem. In exploring the extent to which these substances are used, it is also possible to evaluate the scale of the health risks facing athletes. Based on a review of the available evidence, McDuff et al. (2019) determined that cannabis and cocaine use among athletes was low, as was the rate of substance use disorders in athletes. The review also demonstrated that recreational drug use was longitudinally associated with sporting culture, situational availability, tolerant attitudes among peers and sensation-seeking personality. Reducing recreational drug use therefore requires addressing sociocultural pressures as well as drug testing. Similarly, Docter et al. (2020) examined studies reporting the use of cannabis by athletes and the effects of cannabis on their performance. From a combined sample of 11 studies totalling 46,202 athletes ranging from school to elite level, Docter et al. concluded that one in four (23.4%) athletes had used cannabis in the past 12 months. Furthermore, Docter et al. (2020) stated that 'there was no clearly demonstrated benefit of cannabis use on athletic performance' (p. 197). The conclusion creates a conundrum for regulators as a considerable proportion of the athletic population appear to use cannabis, but do not gain any noticeable performance advantages.

Critics of WADA's prohibition of recreational drugs have argued that banning substances with no performance-enhancing effect, such as marijuana, redefines doping in a way that is no longer concerned with cheating. Instead, WADA is seeking to control an athlete's civic behaviour (Waddington & Møller, 2014, 2019; Waddington et al., 2013). To understand how doping was redefined, it is necessary to return to the original criteria for banning a substance. Prohibition of recreational drugs is a relatively new phenomenon that emerged in the late 1980s and 1990s. In this period, national governments pressured sports organisations to test athletes for recreational drugs in order to protect the image of sport (Waddington et al., 2013). PEDs were previously banned for being performance enhancing and detrimental to athlete welfare. The lack of quality evidence to prove that recreational drugs satisfied either of these conditions meant that sports administrators devised new reasons to prohibit recreational drugs, such as violating the spirit of sport (Waddington et al., 2013). The outcomes of prohibiting substances with an inconsistent rationale, like the spirit of sport, are that disciplinary sanctions for using recreational drugs can be perceived as unjust, sanctions ignore athlete welfare and banning such substances does not stop 'real' cheats. These rationales undermine the legitimacy of WADA because the sanctions are 'irrelevant to the fairness of sporting competition' (Waddington & Møller, 2014, p. 254). Supporting this point, Waddington and Møller (2019) suggested that athletes expect fairness in the anti-doping system, including the treatment of recreational drugs, which is evident in Guerrero's case, as will be discussed later.

Another criticism of prohibiting recreational drugs is that it entrenches the zero-tolerance, punitive approach of the anti-doping system under WADA's control, further stigmatising drug users and neglecting athletes who may require support or treatment (Kayser & O'Hare, 2013). Instead, recreational drugs could be treated as a welfare issue with a policy focused on minimising harm to the athlete. For example, on the point of athlete welfare, one examination of the Australian Football League's Illicit Drug Policy underscored the utility of a harm minimisation approach to recreational drugs management (Harcourt, Unglik, & Cook, 2012). Although testing was conducted out-of-competition as opposed to in-competition, the Illicit Drug Policy prioritised athlete welfare by applying education, counselling, treatment and rehabilitation above ineligibility sanctions. The analysis of the Illicit Drug Policy demonstrated a decrease in positive tests for recreational substances over seven years, during the same period that testing increased by 350% (472 tests in 2005 to 1,489 tests in 2011). The Australian Football League provided proof that harm minimisation, whether it is pursued due to altruism or protecting the brand of a sport, is a feasible alternative to regulating recreational drugs. Dunn (2013) summarised the next challenge if WADA was to pursue a harm minimisation philosophy in observing, 'If we "decriminalise" recreational substance use in sport, what safety nets do we have in place for those athletes who choose to use and whose use becomes problematic' (p. 65)?

Further confounding the ethical and social debate about the status of recreational substances, Heuberger and Cohen (2019) provided a review of the performance-enhancing effects of WADA-prohibited drug groups. They used evidence only from double-blind, randomised controlled trials, considered the gold standard in experimental research design. They also limited studies to experimental designs that used trained subjects (i.e., athletes) and relevant performance outcomes (e.g., aerobic capacity in runners) to ensure transfer to elite sport. Regarding the recreational drug classes banned in-competition, there was no evidence found of performance enhancement from cannabinoids and narcotics, and very limited or mixed evidence regarding stimulants. Regarding cocaine, there was no available evidence from double-blind, randomised controlled trials to determine if it produces relevant ergogenic effects in athletes. Considering that testing for recreational drugs draws away resources from other tasks that may detect athletes using proven PEDs and is complicated by the imperative of discerning whether the athlete used the substance in-competition or OOC, recreational drug prohibition presents a potential black hole for limited resources. The lack of evidence for performance enhancement and testing costs does not mean that recreational drugs should be legalised, but it does place further pressure on other reasons for their prohibition.

Previous discussions of WADA's recreational drug policy and criteria for prohibiting a substance or method reveal that the policy is a source of legitimacy challenges. By including the spirit of sport as a central assessment criterion, WADA has introduced greater subjectivity into the process of prohibiting a substance. This is compounded by the absence of evidence suggesting recreational drugs offer any performance-enhancing effect, therefore giving sanctions a distinct sense of unfairness. The following section will discuss the case of Paolo Guerrero to illustrate the issues with the prohibition of recreational drugs and how these lead to challenges for WADA.

Coca tea, Paolo Guerrero and the World Cup

The case of Guerrero was chosen to exemplify the problems associated with banning recreational drugs and the legitimacy challenges this creates because (1) the high-profile nature of the football World Cup generated widespread coverage globally; (2) the case led to significant actors in the field of anti-doping becoming involved, such as FIFPro (the global professional football player union); (3) it clearly demonstrates the issues discussed in the previous section; and (4) it is a contemporary case. In reviewing the example of Guerrero, we established that he had no intention to enhance his performance, and did not consume the substance in-competition, yet still received a 14-month ban because of the strict liability rule and cocaine's status as a *non-specified substance* (a non-specified substance is less likely to have a credible, non-doping explanation and is subject to stricter sanctions).

On October 5, 2017, Jose Paolo Guerrero, Peruvian national football team captain and Peru's leading goal scorer, provided a doping control sample after a World Cup qualifying match against Argentina that produced an adverse analytical finding for the cocaine metabolite benzoylecgonine. On November 3, the Peruvian Football Federation was informed by FIFA that Guerrero was provisionally suspended for 30 days as cocaine and its analogues are prohibited in-competition under the class of stimulants. This meant that Guerrero, a player described as irreplaceable and the 'soul of the team', was unavailable for Peru's playoff fixtures against New Zealand to qualify for the 2018 World Cup. Despite this setback, for the first time since 1982, Peru qualified for the tournament finals that were to be held in Russia in the following June with a 2-0 aggregate win over New Zealand. The victory placed further pressure for Guerrero's case to be heard in front of FIFA's disciplinary committee at the end of November. On December 7, the disciplinary committee decided that Guerrero should serve a

12-month suspension for the anti-doping rule violation (ADRV). The decision was informed in accordance with the principle of strict liability placed on athletes, which stipulates that all athletes are responsible for any substance found in samples provided, intentional or otherwise (barring exceptional cases).

After Guerrero's appeal to FIFA that the benzoylecgonine was a result of consuming contaminated tea in the team hotel, a claim supported by the low concentration of benzoylecgonine in his sample, the FIFA appeals committee reduced the suspension to six months. The FIFA appeals committee explained the reduction: 'After taking into account all the circumstances of the case, in particular the degree of fault of the player, considered a six-month period of ineligibility to be a proportionate sanction' (FIFA, 2017). With the suspension backdated to November 3 when Guerrero was provisionally suspended, he was now eligible to play in the World Cup in June.

Following the verdict, WADA made the decision to appeal Guerrero's case to CAS in Switzerland and argued for a longer sanction of up to two years. Most recreational drugs are listed as *specified substances* (i.e., less likely to be used for performance enhancement). Despite a lack of evidence to support that cocaine has a performance-enhancing effect, it was listed as a *non-specified substance*. There is less flexibility in reducing punishments for non-specified substances, and therefore there was less lenience available to the arbitrators adjudicating on Guerrero's case. Guerrero also appealed his sentence to CAS with the purpose of having his sanction totally withdrawn. The appeals were heard at the start of May, and as the outcome of the hearing was being determined, Guerrero's six-month suspension expired, which led to him being named in Peru's World Cup squad and representing his club side, the Brazilian team Flamengo. Yet on May 14, 2018, 10 days after the six-month suspension finished, CAS released its decision supporting WADA's appeal and increasing his suspension to 14 months. CAS's decision hinged on the judgement that Guerrero could have made greater efforts to check what tea he was consuming at the team hotel. Therefore, he bore some degree of fault, not *no fault or negligence*. CAS added a suite of actions that Guerrero could have personally taken to reduce the degree of fault:

> There were a number of ways in which Mr Guerrero could, instead of relying on assumptions, have discharged his primary personal duty as an athlete to ensure that no prohibited substance entered his body. He could have inquired as to what protocols operated and where in the hotel. He could have asked specifically what teabags had been put in the jug or jugs in T2 [second cup of tea]. He could have insisted on having the bags brought to him so that he could scrutinize the label (as he claimed to have done with T1 [first cup of tea]) and himself carry out or at least supervise the infusion of the tea. The Panel finds unassailable the decision of the FIFA Disciplinary Committee (endorsed by the FIFA Appeal Committee) that it is not possible to describe Mr Guerrero as being guilty of NFN [no fault or negligence].
>
> (CAS, 2018, p. 18)

Appreciating that athletes should be aware that under strict liability they are responsible for any substance in their bodies and should therefore take precautions, the CAS list of suggestions includes some extreme expectations placed on athletes to verify their food and drink. It is even more illuminating that the CAS decision stated that it 'could entertain with some sympathy' (CAS, 2018, p. 19) a shortened suspension, as Guerrero did not intend to cheat, would not have gained any performance enhancement and an increased ban would stop him captaining Peru at the World Cup. However, CAS then went on to explain that a shortened decision could not be considered as the arbitrators were constrained by the WADC and FIFA's anti-doping regulations, and were therefore compelled to sentence Guerrero to between one and two years.

The perceived unfairness of the decision owing to Guerrero's intent did not go unnoticed and stimulated criticisms of WADA's policy from athletes and sports organisations. Most notably, the player union for professional footballers, FIFPro, stated:

> Both FIFA and the Court of Arbitration for Sport agreed Guerrero did not knowingly ingest the substance and that there was no performance-enhancing effect... It therefore defies common sense that he should be handed a punishment which is so damaging to his career.
>
> (Panja, 2018)

Furthermore, FIFPro sought an urgent meeting with FIFA to discuss changes that would 'protect the fundamental rights of players' (Associated Press, 2018). FIFPro representative Carlos Gonzales directly challenged WADA's policy highlighting the unfairness: 'The paradoxical and absurd thing is that at this time someone who tested positive is competing in the Giro d'Italia' (LatinX Today, 2018). FIFPro also castigated the WADC arguing that Guerrero was 'the latest example of a World Anti-Doping Code that too often leads to inappropriate sanctions, especially when it has been established that there was no intent to cheat' (Homewood, 2018). Gleaves and Christiansen (2019) illustrated the unfairness perceived by many footballers via the online argument between Danish football captain Simon Kjær, who was backed by the Danish Players' Union supporting Guerrero, and Anti Doping Denmark CEO, Michael Ask, who agreed with Guerrero's sanction.

Guerrero subsequently appealed CAS' decision to a Swiss Federal Tribunal. Demonstrating that sport cannot be separated from politics and the importance of Peru's appearance at the World Cup, Peruvian president Martin Vizcarra declared that the Peruvian embassy in Switzerland would 'support the initiatives of the defence of Guerrero before the Swiss federal court to overturn the suspension' (The National, 2018). As Guerrero waited for his opportunity to appeal for a temporary stay on his suspension so that he could play in the World Cup, he received support from his potential World Cup opposition. The captains of the Australian, French and Danish football teams, that Peru was set to play, symbolically co-signed a letter to FIFA requesting that Guerrero be allowed to participate. Other professional footballers in the same period also offered their support for Guerrero due to the perceived unfair suspension (CE Noticias Financieras English, 2018a). UK Anti-Doping (UKAD) Agency chief, Nicole Sapstead, also challenged WADA on its position on recreational drugs. Sapstead argued that recreational drugs do not enhance performance and that a re-evaluation of WADA's policy in determining prohibited substances was required. She contended: 'It is UKAD's view that performance enhancing should be a determining factor - or at least it should fulfil that criterion and then one of the other two' (Slater, 2018). Guerrero's high-profile case functioned as a jolt to bring WADA's legitimacy under debate.

On May 31, Swiss Supreme Court judge Christina Kiss ruled that Guerrero could participate at the World Cup and start his sanction afterwards. Important to this decision was that CAS had already decided that there was no performance-enhancing intent in his behaviour. Consequently, CAS did not challenge the decision to temporarily suspend the sanction (Panja, 2018, May 31). FIFPro reiterated their satisfaction with the decision but also added, 'Along with many professional footballers around the world, we strongly believe that Guerrero's 14-month sanction for unknowingly ingesting a banned substance is unfair and disproportionate' (Gonzalez, 2018), and reiterated the need for reviewing the rules. Despite the seemingly widespread support for Guerrero, some footballers were disappointed at the decision because he had still committed an ADRV (CE Noticias Financieras English, 2018b). Guerrero's case demonstrated how, under the 2015 edition of the WADC, even with no intent to cheat or enhance performance, he still received a 14-month ban. The stress placed on Guerrero going through the judicial process should also be acknowledged, as he highlighted the strain the case placed on both himself and his family, as well as the stigma of being deemed a drug cheat (CE Noticias Financieras English, 2017). Even under the latest rules in the 2021 WADC, Guerrero's ban would have been three months, or potentially one month, if he agreed to attend an approved 'substance of abuse treatment program' (WADC, 2020, p. 66). The question remains, however, given the unfairness of the decision and the stress placed on the athlete, why should an athlete serve a three-month ban or even a one-month ban for drinking a cup of tea? The final section of this chapter will examine how WADA has responded in the revised 2021 WADC to the legitimacy challenges posed by recreational drug prohibition.

Changes in WADA policy

To update the WADC, WADA undertakes a review process with stakeholders that enables them to raise issues they consider need updating or improving. The sanctioning of recreational drugs, and in-particular cocaine, was a significant concern of stakeholders (WADA, 2019). In response, article 10.2.4.1 of the

WADC pertaining to anti-doping rule violations involving a substance of abuse was revised to stipulate:

> If the Athlete can establish that any ingestion or Use occurred Out-of-Competition and was unrelated to sport performance, then the period of Ineligibility shall be three (3) months Ineligibility. In addition, the period of Ineligibility calculated under this Article 10.2.4.1 may be reduced to one (1) month if the Athlete or other Person satisfactorily completes a Substance of Abuse treatment program approved by the Anti-Doping Organization with Results Management responsibility. The period of Ineligibility established in this Article 10.2.4.1 is not subject to any reduction based on any provision in Article 10.6
>
> (WADC, 2020, p. 66).

The revision offered an improvement on the previous situation where athletes could receive up to a two-year ban depending on the substance. WADA's response to the concerns raised about sanctioning recreational drugs, demonstrated by the Guerrero case, fails to stand up to scrutiny when compared to recreational drugs policies of other professional sports. For example, a comparison can be made with the National Football League and Major League Baseball in the United States, which are not signatories to the WADC and determine their own policies. Through collective bargaining with the Players Association, the National Football League announced that substances of abuse are still prohibited because they are detrimental to the welfare of players, but the athletes must now enter an intervention program should they test positive for a substance of abuse (Coffey, 2020). Financial penalties and period of ineligibility sanctions then follow if the athlete does not comply with the intervention program or tests positive again. The emphasis in the National Football League's policy is on player welfare, not punishment. Likewise, Major League Baseball tests for drugs of abuse but adopts a treatment-based approach to positive tests rather than a punitive approach (Major League Baseball Players Association, 2019).

Evidently there is a precedent for a health-focused, harm minimisation approach to recreational drug policies as demonstrated by two of the largest sporting leagues in the world [that do not rely on IOC funding]. Research supports that a harm minimisation approach to recreational drugs might also reduce usage (e.g., Harcourt et al., 2012). The latest WADC stipulating one- to three-month suspensions still seems out of touch with more progressive policies in sport. This position is indicative of the restrictions placed on WADA's capacity for change. As an organisation, WADA functions as part of the wider Olympic movement (Lenskyj, 2020). The organisation's closeness to the Olympic movement is demonstrated symbolically by the importance placed on the spirit of sport, which is termed the 'essence of Olympism' in the WADC (WADC, 2020, p. 13). The relationship between the IOC and WADA undoubtedly influences anti-doping policy direction as it reflects the priorities and principles of the Olympic movement (Read et al., 2019). WADA's recreational drug policy mirrors the IOC's prioritisation of the Summer and Winter Olympic Games' commercial appeal (Lenskyj, 2020) and the seemingly cautious attitude of sponsors towards athletes who use recreational drugs (e.g., the aforementioned example of Phelps losing his contract with Kellogg's).

In revising the WADC, WADA had the opportunity to redefine how recreational drugs are treated by adopting a harm minimisation approach for cases that can be demonstrated to have been out-of-competition and that provided no ergogenic effect, as seen in other policies like the NFL. Instead, the current policy upholds the perspective that athletes are role models who can be used to promote healthy behaviours and appeal to sponsors looking for clean living examples to endorse their products. WADA's capability to respond to legitimacy challenges is restricted to incremental rather than radical change; WADA can make changes in response to legitimacy challenges, but only those changes that maintain the underpinning view of the Olympic movement, and not those demanding a fundamental re-evaluation of the anti-doping philosophy. A switch to a policy direction closer to harm minimisation that treats recreational drug use as a health issue would be in opposition to the morality-based spirit of sport, which currently guides anti-doping efforts under WADA. The outcome is that cases such as that of Paolo Guerrero, where athletes who have not cheated in the typical sense of doping or disadvantaged any opponent (Waddington et al., 2013), will continue to be collateral damage, albeit for a shorter period of ineligibility.

WADA's relationship with national governments also complicates the likelihood of a change in attitudes towards recreational drugs. Despite comments from various heads of national anti-doping agencies about the need for re-evaluation of how recreational drug use is treated (Stuff, 2019), any reduction is likely to be met by stern opposition from government representatives in WADA's Executive Committee and Foundation Board. Large-scale investment into elite sport is commonly justified by governments who use a trickle-down or virtuous cycle of sport argument (Green, 2007; Grix & Carmichael, 2012). The virtuous cycle of sport argument proposes that successful elite athletes function as role models to encourage the general population to exercise and participate in sport. Therefore, investment in elite sport has a net benefit by indirectly encouraging the general population to exercise more. A move towards a recreational drug policy that focuses on welfare rather than punishment may have the double effect of governments: (1) being perceived as going 'soft' on drug use and (2) threatening the role model value of elite athletes. Reflecting on both the pressures from the Olympic movement and national governments, WADA is severely inhibited in how it can respond to the legitimacy challenges arising from recreational drugs. Consequently, an athlete-centred harm minimisation approach seems unlikely.

Conclusion

In conclusion, Guerrero's case exemplified the legitimacy challenges created by WADA's recreational drug policy. That an athlete can demonstrate that he or she did not gain any ergogenic benefit from a substance taken out-of-competition by mistake, and still receives a 14-month suspension, contradicts WADA's ambitions of protecting athletes but exemplifies how WADA's design may lead to stakeholder prioritisation. It was only due to exceptional circumstances and intervention that Guerrero was permitted to compete at the World Cup, the crowning achievement of his career that he might have potentially missed. WADA has shown some flexibility in response to the legitimacy challenges stemming from its recreational drug policy. However, the Guerrero case demonstrates that WADA's capacity for change is limited due to the design and philosophical inflexibility of the organisation's decision-making bodies. Ultimately, WADA had an opportunity to adopt a progressive, athlete-centred policy that promoted welfare rather than punishment. Yet the 2021 WADC reinforces a prohibition approach. As we will discuss in chapter 10, WADA's legitimacy is vulnerable due to its design, and this has implications for how it manages legitimacy challenges. In closing, the problem of recreational drugs is not likely to disappear anytime soon as countries continue to adopt more liberal, health-based policies towards drug use. As more cases, such as Guerrero's, continue to transpire, more pressure will mount on WADA to reconsider its approach to recreational drugs and include athletes in these discussions.

References

Associated Press. (2018). *After Guerrero's World Cup ban, union seeks new doping rules.* Associated Press. Retrieved from https://apnews.com/.

Bergamaschi, M.M., & Crippa, J.A.S. (2013). Why should Cannabis be Considered Doping in Sports? *Frontiers in Psychiatry,* 10.3389/fpsyt.2013.00032.

CAS. (2018). Arbitrations CAS 2018/A/5546 José Paolo Guerrero v. Fédération Internationale de Football Association (FIFA) & CAS 2018/A/5571 World Anti-Doping Agency (WADA) v. FIFA & José Paolo Guerrero, award of 30 July 2018 (operative part of 14 May 2018). Retrieved from http://jurisprudence.tas-cas.org/Help/Home.aspx.

CE *Noticias Financieras English.* (2017). Guerrero after the sanction: I can believe in the injustice that I'm going. Retrieved from Nexis.com.

CE *Noticias Financieras English.* (2018a). Suárez and Godín join in support of Paolo Guerrero. Retrieved from Nexis.com.

CE Noticias Financieras English. (2018b). Captain of Sweden criticizes Guerrero: 'It's sad that if he tested positive, he could play the World Cup'. Retrieved from Nexis.com.

Coffey, G. (2020). Is the NFL removing suspensions for positive drug tests? *Sportscasting.* Retrieved from https://www.sportscasting.com/.

Crean, R.D., Crane, N.A., & Mason, B.J. (2011). An evidence based review of acute and long-term effects of cannabis use on executive cognitive functions. *Journal of Addiction Medicine,* 5(1), 1.

Docter, S., Khan, M., Gohal, C., Ravi, B., Bhandari, M., Gandhi, R., & Leroux, T. (2020). Cannabis use and sport: A systematic review. *Sports Health*, *12*(2), 189–199.

Dunn, M. (2013). Commentary: Ending the ban on recreational substance use in sport: And then what? *Performance Enhancement & Health*, *2*(2), 64–65.

Felson, J., Adamczyk, A., & Thomas, C. (2019). How and why have attitudes about cannabis legalization changed so much? *Social Science Research*, *78*, 12–27.

FIFA. (2017). FIFA Appeal Committee reduces the sanction imposed on Paolo Guerrero to a six-month suspension. FIFA. Retrieved from https://www.fifa.com/.

Gleaves, J., & Christiansen, A.V. (2019). Athletes' perspectives on WADA and the code: A review and analysis. *International Journal of Sport Policy and Politics*, *11*(2), 341–353.

Gonzalez, R. (2018). Peru receives massive boost ahead of World Cup as star striker Guerrero gets special exemption to play. CBS. Retrieved from https://www.cbssports.com/.

Green, M. (2007). Olympic glory or grassroots development?: Sport policy priorities in Australia, Canada and the United Kingdom, 1960–2006. *The International Journal of the History of Sport*, *24*(7), 921–953.

Grix, J., & Carmichael, F. (2012). Why do governments invest in elite sport? A polemic. *International Journal of Sport Policy and Politics*, *4*(1), 73–90.

Harcourt, P.R., Unglik, H., & Cook, J.L. (2012). A strategy to reduce illicit drug use is effective in elite Australian football. *British Journal of Sports Medicine*, *46*(13), 943–945.

Henne, K., Koh, B., & McDermott, V. (2013). Coherence of drug policy in sports: Illicit inclusions and illegal inconsistencies. *Performance Enhancement & Health*, *2*(2), 48–55.

Heuberger, J.A., & Cohen, A.F. (2019). Review of WADA prohibited substances: Limited evidence for performance-enhancing effects. *Sports Medicine*, *49*(4), 525–539.

Homewood, B. (2018). Players' union says Guerrero doping ban defies common sense. *Reuters*. Retrieved from https://uk.reuters.com/.

Huestis, M.A., Mazzoni, I., & Rabin, O. (2011). Cannabis in sport. *Sports Medicine*, *41*(11), 949–966.

International Network of Humanistic Doping Research. (2013). INHDR statement on regulating non-performance enhancing drugs in sport. *Performance Enhancement & Health*, *2*(2), 39–40.

Kayser, B., & O'Hare, P. (2013). Flawed reasoning for testing for recreational drugs in anti-doping. *Performance Enhancement and Health*, *2*(2), 68–69.

LatinX Today. (2018). FIFPro: Guerrero could appeal to Swiss courts to play in World Cup. http://www.latinxtoday.com/.

Lenskyj, H.J. (2020). *The Olympic Games: A critical approach*. Bingley, UK: Emerald Group Publishing.

Lentillon-Kaestner, V. (2013). Should WADA remove the illicit drugs from the prohibited list? *Performance Enhancement & Health*, *2*(2), 70–71.

Macur, J. (2009). Phelps disciplined over marijuana pipe incident. *The New York Times*.

Major League Baseball Players Association. (2019). MLB, MLBPA agree to changes to joint drug program: Parties make significant updates to the drug of abuse provisions of the program. *Major League Baseball Players Association*. Retrieved from https://www.mlbplayers.com/.

McDuff, D., Stull, T., Castaldelli-Maia, J.M., Hitchcock, M.E., Hainline, B., & Reardon, C.L. (2019). Recreational and ergogenic substance use and substance use disorders in elite athletes: A narrative review. *British Journal of Sports Medicine, 53*(12), 754–760.

McNamee, M.J. (2012). The spirit of sport and the medicalisation of anti-doping: Empirical and normative ethics. *Asian Bioethics Review, 4*(4), 374–392.

The National. (2018). President of Peru backs captain Paolo Guerrero over World Cup doping ban. Retrieved from https://www.thenational.ae/.

Panja, T. (2018). Peru's Paolo Guerrero vows to fight doping ban: 'This is about my honor'. *The New York Times.*

Read, D, Skinner, J, Lock, D, & Houlihan, B (2019). Legitimacy driven change at the World Anti-Doping Agency. *International Journal of Sport Policy and Politics,* 11, 233–245. 10.1080/19406940.2018.1544580.

Saugy, M., Avois, L., Saudan, C., Robinson, N., Giroud, C., Mangin, P., & Dvorak, J. (2006). Cannabis and sport. *British Journal of Sports Medicine, 40,* 13–15.

Slater, M. (2018). UKAD calls on WADA to clarify cocaine policy as Paolo Guerrero appeals to FIFA. *The Press Association.*

Stuff. (2019). Bans for recreational drugs could be reduced to four weeks under new Wada code. *Stuff.* Retrieved from https://www.stuff.co.nz/.

WADA. (2019). Minutes of the WADA Executive Committee Meeting 15 May 2019, Montreal, Canada: WADA. Retrieved from https://www.wada-ama.org/.

WADC. (2020). World Anti-Doping Code 2021. Retrieved from https://www.wada-ama.org/.

Waddington, I., Christiansen, A.V., Gleaves, J., Hoberman, J., & Møller, V. (2013). Recreational drug use and sport: Time for a WADA rethink?. *Performance Enhancement & Health, 2*(2), 41–47.

Waddington, I., & Møller, V. (2014). Cannabis use and the spirit of sport: A response to Mike McNamee. *Asian Bioethics Review, 6*(3), 246–258.

Waddington, I., & Møller, V. (2019). WADA at twenty: Old problems and old thinking? *International Journal of Sport Policy and Politics, 11*(2), 219–231.

Chapter 9

The Russian Olympic doping scandal

It is evident from the preceding case studies that the field of Olympic sport is characterised by a diverse range of stakeholders with their own political and commercial agendas, which are often intertwined. The International Olympic Committee (IOC) has always claimed to be apolitical and, therefore, does not involve itself in global diplomatic affairs. The Olympics are instead portrayed as events that can rise above political tensions and unite the world. The reality is somewhat less idealistic as, despite the IOC's best attempts, the history of the Olympic Games is littered with political boycotts, protests and controversies. As recently as the 2018 PyeongChang Winter Olympics, the IOC found itself trying to navigate the long-running diplomatic frictions between South Korea, North Korea and the United States. Historically anti-doping regulation has also been unable to avoid the partisan nature of elite international sports and associated geo-political tensions. The final case study presented in this chapter focuses on the exposure of the systematic doping programme in Russia that involved more than 1,000 athletes across multiple Olympic and international sporting events. Reminiscent of the state-implemented doping programme of East Germany during the Cold War, the Russian doping scandal was widely considered as the most significant doping scandal to occur during World Anti-Doping Agency's (WADA) existence, spurring a range of issues for WADA (e.g., the Fancy Bears data leak discussed in chapter six).

The exposure of a systematic doping programme in Russia demonstrated how anti-doping testing could be systematically evaded on a national scale at the Olympic Games through manipulation of doping control samples. The revelations also exposed a reluctance from a number of key stakeholders in sport, including WADA and the IOC, to acknowledge the problem of doping due to commercial implications. The significance of systematic doping in Russia was heightened by the fact that it was situated in the larger geo-political role of international sport. Sport has always functioned as an arena for national rivals to exercise their power through dominance of the Olympic medal tables at great economic cost. A dynamic that has been further complicated by the emergence of China as a sporting superpower. Given the value governments place on demonstrating sporting prowess as a proxy of national and military status, the indication of a systematic, national doping programme in Russia could be framed as an attack on the political ambitions of rival nations.

As a consequence of sport's prominence in a larger international power contest, WADA found itself not only as the global regulator of doping but also as an arbitrator of geo-political tensions. Recognising its position, every decision WADA made regarding anti-doping efforts in Russia has been subject to complex commercial and political pressures. Accordingly, WADA's legitimacy was subject to scrutiny and challenge from a diverse array of stakeholders throughout the Russian scandal, providing an opportunity to develop our understanding of the current consensus around WADA within the field of anti-doping. To examine the diversity of propriety judgements expressed during the Russian Olympic doping scandal, this chapter is structured as follows. Firstly, a timeline is provided from the exposure of Russian doping in 2014 via a documentary from German media company ARD through to the 2018 PyeongChang Winter Olympics and WADA's ongoing management of Russia's compliance status in 2020. The purpose of the timeline is to familiarise the reader with how the scandal unfolded and identify how WADA's legitimacy was challenged and by whom during the course of the scandal. Secondly, three key themes are discussed in relation to the legitimacy processes around WADA in this period: (1) WADA was subject to conflicting expectations of legitimate behaviour from two groups, inter-governmental community and sport governing bodies; (2) WADA's behavioural response to challenges was reactive in the form of 'legitimacy-driven change' to ensure organisational survival; and (3) WADA relied on a rhetoric of success, avoiding admission of wrongdoing. The chapter finishes by concluding on the case in connection to the previous case studies.

The Russian Olympic doping scandal timeline

There are a series of critical periods related to the Russian doping scandal drawn out over six years that have encouraged challenges to WADA's legitimacy. These events are now described in chronological order, detailing the sources of challenge to WADA and how they developed over time.

On December 3, 2014, using information from whistle-blowers Yuliya Stepanova, a Russian athlete, and Vitaly Stepanov, a Russian anti-doping agency employee, German journalist Hajo Seppelt presented a documentary broadcast on ARD media accusing the All-Russian Athletic Federation (ARAF) of a systematic doping programme. Following the documentary being aired, challenges to WADA were predominantly limited to journalists covering the story as both WADA and the IOC looked to World Athletics (formerly the IAAF) to take the lead ('Majority of Russian athletes', 1). At this point, the only legitimacy challenges to WADA were based on the perceived inadequacy of testing from journalists to whom the organisation had little accountability. In response, WADA launched what would be the first of two investigations into alleged doping violations in Russia.

The first investigation was led by former WADA President and IOC member Dick Pound, the results of which were published in two parts. Part one was published on November 9, 2015, and documented bribery and corruption within World Athletics and the ARAF related to covering up failed anti-doping tests (Pound, McLaren, & Younger, 2). The second investigation, published on January 14, 2016, supported these findings with additional evidence (Pound, McLaren, & Younger, 3). The two reports did little to provoke further challenges to WADA's legitimacy, with stakeholders instead focused on World Athletics' failings. In some instances, the willingness of WADA to investigate even drew positive evaluations (iNADO, 4). WADA did, however, attract negative attention in the interim between the reports due to a leaked memo from WADA President Sir Craig Reedie to staff in November 2015. Reedie suggested in the memo that WADA's response to Seppelt's documentary and Russian doping should be based on the severity of public reaction. Some critics interpreted Reedie's memo to mean that WADA may not have acted had Russia's behaviour been less widely condemned (Walsh, 5, November 8). The memo was a catalyst leading to challenges, more so than the original documentary, but criticisms of WADA's willingness to detect and punish doping were again limited to journalists.

The leaked memo was reinforced in early May 2016 by two separate interviews conducted in the United States with whistle-blower Vitaly Stepanov and the former Russian Anti-Doping Agency (RUSADA) director Grigory Rodchenkov. The interviewees alleged that the anti-doping laboratory at the 2014 Sochi Winter Olympic Games had been corrupted by the Russian government and that WADA had failed to act on information provided to them about Russian doping as early as 2010. These revelations drew in organisations that openly questioned WADA's commitment, as a chorus of athletes, national governments and National Anti-Doping Organisations (NADOs) all used the information to dispute WADA's intent to stop doping.

In light of the interviews and subsequent challenges, WADA funded a second investigation into Russian doping headed by Canadian lawyer Richard McLaren. The first McLaren (2016a) report concluded that (a) 'the Moscow Laboratory operated, for the protection of doped Russian athletes, within a State-dictated failsafe system' (p. 1) controlled by the Ministry of Sport and (b) 'the Sochi Laboratory operated a unique sample swapping methodology to enable doped Russian athletes to compete at the Games' (p. 1). The report brought to the fore geo-political questions about anti-doping. Given the similarities between Russian doping and the doping activities of the former Soviet Union (Kalinski, 7), the Russian doping scandal fitted into a wider narrative of the modern cold war in sport, where athletes of superpower nations function as foot soldiers (Altukhov & Nauright, 8). The first McLaren report was controversially delivered three weeks before the 2016 Rio Olympics, accompanied by a suggestion from WADA to ban all Russian athletes from participating at the upcoming Olympic Games. WADA's suggestion created significant attention and debate about the organisation's legitimacy. By calling for a blanket ban, WADA positioned itself with groups that had previously challenged its legitimacy. In this sense, WADA demonstrated the same shared judgements of propriety as vocal athletes, national governments and NADOs; namely, that there should be zero tolerance to doping. However, in positioning itself as an investigator and judge, rather than just a regulatory agency, it drew challenges from the IOC and other IFs who constituted a major source of historical legitimacy for WADA. The questions WADA had previously faced for not investigating Russian doping sooner were elevated by IOC officials to challenge WADA's very existence. These tensions in the relationship between WADA and the IOC continued until a proverbial ceasefire was agreed between the leaders of the two organisations in May 2017 (IOC, 2017a).

Ultimately, the IOC allowed each IF to determine whether there should be Russian participation in the Olympic Games, arguing that collective responsibility was unfair. The decision created a rift between WADA and the IOC. Savulescu (2016)10 discussed the blanket ban for Russian athletes from a 'standards of guilt' perspective. The result of his philosophical thought experiment indicated that collective responsibility was not fair to athletes. Restricting athletes of their basic liberty to work (i.e., compete at the Olympic Games) required evidence beyond reasonable doubt that an athlete had doped, and instead regulatory agencies should bear the consequences of inadequate testing. However, the International Paralympic Committee did ban all Russian athletes from the Rio Paralympic Games. A decision that was subsequently upheld by the Court of Arbitration for Sport (CAS). The McLaren report has since been argued by Girginov and Parry (2018) to have undermined the integrity of sport as well. Their argument was based on the political nature of the decision to investigate Russia, the flawed data collection methodologies, the stark deficiencies in the anti-doping system revealed by the investigation and the new expectation of WADA to investigate all claims for the sake of equality.

In the months following the 2016 Olympic Games, the IOC scrutinised the legitimacy of WADA. In this period, the second McLaren (2016b) report was released, supporting the findings of the first stating that 'over 1000 Russian athletes competing in summer, winter and Paralympic sport, can be identified as being involved in or benefiting from manipulations to conceal positive doping tests' (p. 2). The rift between the IOC and WADA continued until May 2017, when they publicly agreed to reconcile their differences before the 2018 PyeongChang Winter Olympics. The Russian Olympic Committee was suspended from the PyeongChang Games, and Russian athletes who could demonstrate a record of completing anti-doping tests could compete as an 'Olympic athlete from Russia', but the national anthem and flag were prohibited. Although WADA was able to find peace with the IOC after this chaotic period, long-term challenges emerged after the PyeongChang Winter Olympics about how to manage the compliance status of RUSADA.

WADA's handling of RUSADA and Russia's position in the world of international sport led to legitimacy challenges from 2017 to 2020. The suspension of the Russian Olympic Committee at the 2018 PyeongChang Winter Olympics coupled with the presence of Russian athletes under the title of 'Olympic athletes from Russia', drew criticism about the extent to which Russia had been punished. However, the IOC was predominantly the target of this criticism. The major legitimacy challenges for WADA were to follow. In September 2018, WADA drew disapproval from certain stakeholders in the anti-doping field as they decided to reinstate RUSADA as a compliant anti-doping agency. Russia was reinstated despite failing to supply laboratory information management system (LIMS) data from the Moscow laboratory that could be used to investigate individual athletes. The situation was further compounded as RUSADA's reinstatement had rested on the LIMS data being provided by January 1, 2019, a deadline which was subsequently missed. As Dasgupta (2017)13 argued, Russia's position as a sporting elite superpower, furnished with economic and political authority, enables it to exploit the anti-doping system with reduced fear of reprisal from WADA.

When the LIMS data were finally handed over by Russia later in January 2019, under closer inspection it was revealed to have been tampered with, drawing further criticism of WADA's handling of the scandal. In December 2019, the WADA Executive Committee voted to ban Russia from being represented in international sports based on the evidence of data tampering. However, Russian athletes who could demonstrate they were not implicated with doping could still compete under a neutral flag. The ban was criticised by some anti-doping officials for being symbolic rather than substantive. Russia also appealed the decision to CAS with the hope of having it removed. Russia's fate in Olympic sport, and at least to some extent WADA's legitimacy, will be determined by the CAS arbitration in November 2020.

The scale of doping uncovered in Russia has unsurprisingly generated significant commentary on WADA's recent anti-doping efforts and sport's wider role in society. As Hermann (2019)14 noted, given the relative performance of other leading Olympic nations compared to Russia, which was known to be operating a systematic doping programme, either the benefits of doping are overstated or there may be reason to question the integrity of other nations. The scandal provides a unique case of gross non-compliance with the WADC to study how the legitimacy of WADA has been challenged and how WADA has responded. The following section will now discuss the three key points in relation to WADA's legitimacy that have emerged from the analysis of the key events specified: conflicting sources of legitimacy, short-term change and success rhetoric.

Conflicting sources of legitimacy

WADA was subject to 'conflicting sources of legitimacy' as two clear groups of challengers appeared with different expectations of behaviour: (1) the inter-governmental community, and (2) sport-governing bodies. The first group, the inter-governmental community, consisted of NADOs, activist government representatives, journalists and athletes. In assessing the legitimacy of WADA, these evaluators were united by the shared belief that WADA should have greater capabilities regarding monitoring and sanctioning compliance and should be further separated from intrusion by representatives of sport organisations (Gibson, 15, November 11). For example, following the first McLaren report, Canadian Sports Minister Carla Qualtrough suggested that WADA should have greater powers to sanction non-compliance: 'It is imperative that there are consequences at all levels for those who are cheating the system, not just the athletes' (Gillespie, 16, July 19). The second group, sport-governing bodies, dominated by the Olympic movement (the IOC, national Olympic committees and IFs), believed that WADA has a specific and exclusive purpose, and should not be simultaneously responsible for creating policy, monitoring compliance and punishing non-compliance. Spanish Olympic Committee President Alejandro Blanco's rhetorical statement, 'What is WADA for?' (Wilson, 17, November 16), was a critical reference to WADA's handling of, and involvement in, the first McLaren report. As we will go on to demonstrate, the beliefs of this group were at odds with the typical criticisms levied against WADA in the same period of instability.

The inter-governmental group of NADOs, government representatives, journalists and athletes perceived WADA's initial inability to successfully enforce and monitor code compliance, and the apparent apathy demonstrated by the leaked memo, (Walsh, 5, November 8) as reasons to question WADA's legitimacy. *New York Times* journalist Christopher Clarey (2015, December 1) 18 summarised feelings towards the first Pound Report:

> Though it is encouraging that WADA and the IAAF are acting and investigating, it would have been a great deal more convincing if all this had come to light via internal inquiries rather than via external investigations by news organizations.

Similarly, Richard Ings, former Chief Executive of the Australian Anti-Doping Agency argued in response to the publication of the first Pound Report:

> Remember, it was the media, not the system, that picked up these issues. Indeed, the system for some time pushed back on the media message, so any system that allows this type of conduct to occur is a flawed system.
>
> (Clarey, 18, December 1)

Certain athlete groups who have the least representation in WADA (an appointed rather than elected advisory committee), also voiced concerns during this period, perhaps because they had the most to gain from a new organisation. Over 20 athlete groups petitioned WADA, calling on them to investigate the allegations made by Grigory Rodchenkov (Ingle, 2016, June 14). Athlete groups further petitioned for an athlete charter of rights to protect their interests (Beacon, 20, May 19).

Failure to investigate doping issues and demonstrate a willingness to catch cheats was judged as illegitimate behaviour and led to legitimacy challenges. Travis Tygart, head of USADA argued:

> WADA's foot-dragging has raised serious questions about the agency's willingness to do its job. Since it was founded in 2000, the United States Anti-Doping Agency has advocated separation between those who promote sport and those who police it. To do otherwise is to have the fox guarding the henhouse.
>
> (Tygart, 21)

Likewise, anti-doping expert Richard Ings questioned WADA following the McLaren report based on indications that they had not investigated Russia sooner: 'It was all avoidable. Everyone knew there were serious problems with Russia in 2013, yet WADA did nothing until nearly 18 months late' (Ingle, 2016, July 23).

As the Russian Olympic scandal progressed into 2018 with questions about RUSADA's compliance status, WADA began to draw stronger legitimacy challenges from the inter-governmental group that demanded widespread reform of anti-doping. Before RUSADA could be reinstated, the expectations from these stakeholders were consistent that Russia had not publicly accepted the outcomes of the McLaren Investigation or provided access to the Moscow Laboratory and could not be allowed to return until doing so. The Institute for National Anti-Doping Organisations (iNADO) exemplified this position:

> Any reasonable person would conclude that Russia has not yet fulfilled its obligations to the global sporting community. WADA must make its decisions based on consistent application of principles and not simply out of expedience pandering to the will of a powerful nation.
>
> (iNADO, 22a)

When WADA reinstated RUSADA, there was widespread condemnation among governments, athletes and NADOs. WADA Vice-President Linda Helleland, who voted against Russia's reinstatement, emphasized: 'Today we made the wrong decision in protecting the integrity of sport and to maintain public trust. Today we failed clean athletes of the world' ('Athletes failed', 23). Similarly damning, former WADA executive and current Athletics Integrity Unit Chairman, David Howman, stated:

WADA has gone from being an organisation that cared about clean athletes to one that cares about international federations that have not been able to stage events in Russia: it's money over principle. That is quite a difference, quite a swing, from what WADA once was.

('Triumph for money', 24)

After WADA followed the advice of the Compliance Review Committee to reinstate RUSADA, there was widespread dissent among the NADOs, athlete representatives and governments for root-and-branch reform of anti-doping as well. As Travis Tygart proclaimed, 'The road to the new, stronger WADA must start now. And let's be clear: absolutely nothing will be off the table for how we, the anti-doping community, begin the work of reforming WADA' (USADA, 25). Athlete groups, such as GlobalAthlete, began to emerge championing reform, and major NADOs gave their support to the governance reforms being demanded. Support for the reforms culminated in an endorsement from the iNADO, a collection of established NADOs from elite sporting countries (Dasgupta, 13):

Given the athletes' concerns in WADA's decision-making and governance process, and after all that we have regrettably witnessed in the wake of the Russian doping crisis, WADA's limited proposals for governance reform fall far short of what the world's athletes and other champions of clean sport have been calling for these past two years, and there should be a rethink.

(iNADO, 2018b)

Evidently, the inter-governmental group believed that the legitimacy of WADA was vulnerable enough to demand sweeping change. The Russian scandal raises similarities with the Festina affair that led to the creation of WADA, and a sense of deja vu as another high-profile scandal drew governments into further debates about managing anti-doping.

The sport-governing bodies group consisted of representatives from the IOC, national Olympic committees and IFs. The group was characterised by a pragmatic judgement that WADA is a regulatory body and its functions should be limited to this capacity. Any activities outside of a regulatory capacity should be judged as illegitimate, a violation to WADA's mandate and subject to challenge. For example, in discussing responsibility for failing to detect Russian doping, IOC member Gerardo Werthein articulated concerns about WADA's behaviour: 'At times WADA has seemed to be more interested in publicity and self-promotion rather than doing its job as a regulator' ('WADA in the cross-hairs', 26, August 2). Similarly, a press release by the International Swimming Federation (FINA) prior to the McLaren report raised concerns about WADA overstepping its responsibilities: '[FINA] is also concerned that there has been a drive behind the scenes to get a global coalition to support the call for the total ban on Russia' (Lalovic, 2016, July 17). Other IF representatives were also indignant as WADA called for a total ban, as International Gymnastics Federation President Bruno Grandi exemplified: 'Blanket bans have never been and will never be just' (Herman, 28, July 18).

The handling of RUSADA's compliance status appeared to generate less criticism from stakeholders embedded in the Olympic movement, potentially due to the truce agreed between WADA and the IOC (IOC, 2017a). IOC President Thomas Bach regularly supported the autonomy of WADA: 'The IOC in the Olympic Charter has accepted the World Anti-Doping Code, and if there is a decision being issued according to the World Anti-Doping Code, it is mandatory for the IOC' (Maese, 29). That WADA's decisions supported Russian athletes participating in Olympic events – even if under a neutral flag – also aided the financial interests of the Olympic movement as evidenced by the divide in WADA's Executive Committee and the desire to reinstate Russia ('Tensions emerge', 30).

The challenges presented by the sport-governing bodies can be understood by the threat WADA's behaviour posed at the time to the commercial objectives of the Olympic movement. There is an element of this threat in WADA's call for a ban on Russian participation given the revenue and support Russian sponsors and government provide to the IOC and IFs (Weston Phippen, 31, July 28). The IOC was largely uninvolved in the scandal with regards to WADA's behaviour until it posed a commercial threat at Rio 2016. WADA's suggestion of a blanket ban was a threat to the commercial income of the IOC. For example, Russian State Television threatened to withdraw coverage of the 2018 PyeongChang Winter Olympic Games if Russia received a complete ban ('Russian State Television', 32, December 5). The loss of revenue from this market would have been a significant blow to the IOC.

WADA's failings in identifying Russian doping sooner and the suggestion that Russia should be handed a blanket ban were perceived by the IOC Executive Committee and other sporting bodies as WADA overstepping its remit. WADA's job was to regulate and monitor anti-doping policy, not to determine sanctions for non-compliance. Sanctions were the responsibility of the relevant sporting organisation, in this instance the IOC, which then delegated to IFs. For example, at an IOC meeting prior to the Rio Games, Italian IOC member Mario Pescante argued that responsibility for the situation was WADA's fault: 'WADA's failure has left the sports movement in a very difficult position and an impossible time frame' (Slater, 33, August 3). Similarly, following the 2016 Rio Olympic Games, IOC member Gerardo Werthein called for a new IOC integrity unit to manage anti-doping:

> Despite the various inquiries which have been launched, we have still not had an adequate explanation on why WADA did not act earlier on the situation in Russia when they had been fully alerted to the doping problem as early as 2010 ... Nor have we been provided with any serious analysis as to how WADA has let the sports movement and national governments

spend major amounts of money on almost 300,000 tests per year and yet find so few of those who appear now to have been cheating.

(Ingle & Gibson, 34, September 21)

Given that some IF representatives and IOC executives have historically considered WADA to be an inconvenience rather than a solution (Hunt, 2011), challenges are not unexpected.

As previously mentioned, WADA and the IOC agreed to reconcile in 2017 before the PyeongChang Olympics. At the time, members of the Olympic movement were pushing for Russia's reinstatement as soon as possible. For example, at a WADA Foundation Board meeting in May 2018, IOC member Patrick Baumann queried: 'We don't challenge the road map, we simply question for how long we want to follow that road map - for the next 10 years, 20 years, 30 years?' ('Tensions emerge', 30). Accordingly, commentary from members of the Olympic movement was relatively supportive of WADA's decisions in relation to RUSADA because WADA's decisions did not focus on collective punishment of athletes, the same position adopted by the IOC for both Rio de Janeiro and Pyeongchang Olympics (Gleeson, 35). Supporting this perspective, an IOC press statement following the recommendations to sanction WADA for manipulating the LIMS data declared:

> The IOC welcomes the opportunity offered by WADA to Russian athletes to compete, 'where they are able to demonstrate that they are not implicated in any way by the non-compliance'... The IOC emphasises that any sanctions should follow the rules of natural justice and respect human rights. Therefore, the IOC stresses that the guilty should be punished in the toughest way possible because of the seriousness of this infringement and thus welcomes the sanctions for the Russian authorities responsible.
>
> (IOC, 36)

Compared to the Rio Olympics where WADA advocated for a blanket ban, the decision aligned with the IOC's position as it was the Russian Olympic Committee and representatives who shouldered the consequences rather than athletes.

To summarise, throughout the scandal, WADA's legitimacy was divided between two primary groups defined by shared legitimacy criteria: (1) sport-governing bodies and (2) the inter-governmental community. The legitimacy of WADA was further complicated as these sources were relatively inflexible in judging the behaviour of WADA.

Short-term change

Short-term change builds on the notion of conflicting sources of legitimacy because WADA has responded with short-term reactive changes to address immediate legitimacy challenges rather than long-term proactive strategy. Problematically, we argue that WADA devised policy reactively privileging powerful stakeholders that immediate organisational survival depended upon rather than proactively, excluding deeper reflection on policy paradigms.

Our analysis reveals that WADA's anti-doping policy agenda was largely reactive in the sense that it was shaped and modified on the basis of responses to public criticisms and stakeholder demands. For example, since 2016, WADA has expanded its Intelligence and Investigations Department; developed 'Speak Up!', a secure online platform for doping informants; and created a whistle-blower protection policy. It is likely that these changes occurred only because WADA's legitimacy was challenged in relation to its handling of the Stepanovas by the IOC. For example, IOC President Thomas Bach identified WADA's poor whistle-blower protocols as the reason for its decision to allow IFs to decide on Russia's inclusion or exclusion for the 2016 Olympics (Ruiz, 2016, August 1).

The extraordinary summit of NADOs on August 30, 2016 (LawInSport, 38) at which 17 leading NADO's proposed a series of reforms was another example of reactive change. The reforms included transparency in decision-making, increased financial investment, removal of conflicts of interest held by decision makers at WADA, separation of code non-compliance consequences from sport, greater investigative capacities and better protection for whistle-blowers. Calls for independence, transparency and investment were accepted by WADA executives, but not actioned. WADA President, Sir Craig Reedie raised the issue that WADA was underfunded and his successor, Witold Bańka, later highlighted funding as a key area for reform throughout his election campaign. Future WADA presidents will not be able to concurrently serve any role with an IF or national administration, however, the Executive Committee will still be comprised of Olympic movement officials and government representatives. It is unlikely that WADA would have created a governance working group to review management processes before stakeholders publicly targeted the conflict of interest. Finally, graded sanctions for non-compliance have recently been introduced under the ISCCS policy. Again, this was a response to the challenges from government and anti-doping groups about sanctioning Russia over non-compliance. WADA had dedicated most of its time and efforts to remedying issues that stakeholders raised with seemingly little consideration of *why* the problems arose in the first place.

In the five years since the Russian Olympic doping scandal, WADA's agenda has been predominantly determined by responding to the emergent challenges. This is clear in the governance reforms, improved investigative capacity, whistle-blower support policies and International Testing Agency (ITA). Although these reforms were required, they were not coupled with a fundamental re-evaluation of the reasons the problems emerged. The focus has been on "how" systematic doping was able to occur, not "why". Furthermore, the national governments, groups and organisations that have challenged WADA throughout the scandal are from the Olympic sporting elite (Dasgupta, 13). Consequently, the issues experienced by other WADA signatories were sidelined. This is evidenced by the prominence USADA has had throughout the scandal, using America's position as the largest funder of WADA to urge change suiting their agenda. As a global regulator, anti-doping is only as strong as its weakest member, and if WADA pursues reform driven by short-term reactive responses driven by its most powerful stakeholders, then the results may further marginalise the interests of weaker stakeholders.

WADA's responses can also be differentiated by the type of challenge posed and the level of action required. WADA was more likely to address challenges based on pragmatic criteria targeting the organisation's performance. For example, the decision to launch both investigations into Russia reflected consent to performance challenges from sources who demanded that the claims from the ARD documentary and Rodchenkov were investigated in greater detail ('Report details', 2016, May 14). WADA itself was not criticised, and therefore conformity did not require any admission of fault. However, moral challenges or calls for fundamental policy revision by WADA were more likely to be met by symbolic or defiant responses that avoided recognising the arguments put forward. For example, when challenged about the conflict of interests within WADA's structure, Sir Craig Reedie countered: 'This marriage has worked. If people believe there is a conflict of interest, then clearly, I have to deal with that perception' (Waldie, 39, June 20). Reedie's statement simultaneously refuted claims that there was a problem with how WADA was organised and suggested that challenges could be solved by improving public relations rather than through reflection and substantive change.

From an organisational perspective, the responsibility for performance problems can be placed upon the implementation of a policy rather than the policy creator itself. For instance, following the first Pound Report, despite WADA's shortcomings in monitoring RUSADA and preventing the corruption of anti-doping management, blame was attributed to external factors. As Dick Pound stated after the publication of the first Pound Report: 'Our problem was people. Once again, the people broke down, not the system' (Dickinson, 40, November 10). When presented with challenges to WADA's values, such as those posed about the organisation's unwillingness to actively investigate allegations of doping, any form of admission of guilt would undermine the legitimacy of WADA. Defiance and symbolic action become methods of avoiding deep reflection on the performance of the principles and arguments that underpin WADA's anti-doping system.

We argue that short-term change also privileged the stakeholders with the greatest power, defined by the influence they have over WADA. The IOC contributes 50% of WADA's funding, and therefore when the IOC demonstrated a willingness to consider other institutional arrangements regarding anti-doping management (e.g., establishing an IOC integrity unit) following the Rio Olympics, WADA responded with noteworthy changes.

Although it is not known to what degree an IOC Integrity Unit was a serious consideration or just posturing, WADA responded to its concerns with substantive policy change. For example, several IOC members commented on the ability of Russian athletes to evade WADA testing (Ingle & Gibson, 34, September 21). WADA has consequently proceeded with supporting the development of the ITA. An idea originally proposed by the IOC (2017b), the ITA is tasked with implementing testing for sporting organisations to reduce conflicts of interest. The IOC's influence is heightened by their promise of greater funding if WADA created the testing authority ('IOC promises', 42, October 8). However, the promise of supplemental funding for the ITA was criticised by journalists due to the number of IOC members on its Executive Committee. In fact, the committee's composition forced a name change from independent to international as the organisation could not be considered independent (Butler, 2018, March 23). As a result, the IOC has gained further influence over anti-doping policy and testing implementation. Following the end to hostilities between WADA and the IOC, the Olympic movement has been supportive of WADA's decisions regarding RUSADA that avoided sanctioning athletes. There is obvious merit in the argument to avoid sanctioning athletes who can clearly demonstrate that they have not been involved in the Russian doping programme (e.g., foreign-based Russian athletes) and allow them to compete. Critically, WADA's approach may also be a deliberate decision to align with the Olympic movement, its primary funder.

Short-term change was one tactic that WADA used in response to challenges. The tactic was problematic from a policy creation perspective as important issues may be neglected if they are not from a stakeholder perceived as valuable to WADA or do not generate a large media profile. An unwillingness to compromise the values and structure of WADA has constrained WADA's consideration of alternative anti-doping policy directions such as a harm reduction approach or integrated player unions. In contrast to this point, former WADA President Reedie stated in 2018:

> The review of WADA's governance model has been extensive and has clearly shown WADA's willingness to adapt. In an ever-changing world, WADA's role has grown and evolved since its current governance model was first formed. It is right that the structure should develop as well and should continue to be looked at in the future. This should not be thought of as the end of a process but, in fact, it is really the beginning of an ongoing process of governance review within WADA.
>
> (WADA, 2018)

Although the evidence we have presented proves that WADA did adapt when confronted with challenges, its willingness to change was restricted to incremental and tokenistic movements that largely maintained the status quo, rather than any radical shifts to revise platform policy. The final section of this chapter discusses how WADA sought to project an image of success throughout the crisis period.

Success rhetoric

The final theme discussed concerns WADA's 'success rhetoric'. Throughout the scandal, WADA's leaders portrayed it as winning the fight against doping in sport, while also denying any deficiencies or accepting any fault. The rhetoric employed suggested a tendency for WADA to dismiss challenges and maintain its values. Previous research has suggested that the IOC has a history of rhetorically constructing doping in sport as a war they were fighting and winning (Wagner & Pedersen, 43). WADA drew upon this rhetorical tactic by utilising language that implied WADA was in control, had committed no wrongdoing and was successfully combatting doping in sport.

WADA's success rhetoric is evident from the start of the scandal. In launching the Pound investigation, the comments of Sir Craig Reedie suggested an attempt to emphasise that WADA was in control of the situation:

> Once the investigation is concluded, if it is found that there have been violations or breaches of the rules, WADA will ensure that any individuals or organizations concerned are dealt with in an appropriate fashion under the World Anti-Doping Code.
>
> (WADA, 44)

WADA's intention to project a rhetoric of control is evident in specific terms and phrases they used. For example, the term 'ensure' gave WADA a sense that justice for athletes was certain. Similarly, the statement to the press from Sir Craig Reedie after the 2014 Sochi Winter Olympics doping scandal had been exposed presented an image that WADA was in control of the situation by launching the McLaren investigation. WADA also placed fault on Rodchenkov for not releasing information about doping previously:

> WADA will probe these new allegations immediately. The claims made in the program offer real cause for concern, as they contain new allegations regarding attempts to subvert the anti-doping process at the Sochi Game. Mr. Rodchenkov was of course interviewed by WADA's Independent Commission that exposed widespread doping in Russian athletics last year; yet, regrettably, he was not forthcoming with such information related to the Sochi Games. It is surprising to hear these views so many months after the Commission concluded its work.
>
> (WADA, 2016a)

The use of the word 'immediately' gave the launch of the investigation a sense of urgency and proactivity despite it being reactive. Likewise, the language 'of course', and reminder that WADA 'exposed widespread doping in Russian athletics', portrayed the organisation as doing the right things in order to successfully catch doping cheats.

WADA also asserted that it was in a position of control throughout the RUSADA reinstatement process. Reedie used the notion of controlling proceedings to justify the decision: 'This decision provides a clear timeline by which WADA must be given access to the former Moscow laboratory data and samples with a clear commitment by the ExCo that should this timeline not be met, it would support the CRC's [Compliance Review Committee] recommendation to reinstate non-compliance' (WADA, 2018a). By compromising at this stage and agreeing a date for access to the data, WADA was eventually able to gain access after a long deadlock. It is not possible to determine whether the data would have been eventually obtained if RUSADA had not been reinstated. However, it is worth questioning to what extent Russia's prominence in the Olympic movement prompted WADA to compromise, and whether a less important Olympic nation would have been treated the same.

In terms of maintaining an image of no wrongdoing, WADA stood behind procedural arguments when defending itself. For example, WADA's legitimacy was challenged by several stakeholders due to their poor treatment of the Stepanovs. In responding to these challenges, Sir Craig Reedie did not acknowledge any wrongdoing and placed the blame on procedural problems and a lack of power:

> What may have appeared as inaction reflected the fact that, until the revised World Anti-Doping Code came into effect on 1 January 2015, WADA did not have the power to conduct its own investigations. At the time, the Agency was only able to collect information and pass it on to those that did have the power to investigate, in this case, the Russian authorities. WADA believes that passing the whistle-blowers' information on to the Russian authorities would not have resulted in the required scrutiny.
>
> (WADA, 2016a)

It is evident in this quote that Reedie believed WADA was incapable of doing more. WADA also came under fire for its decision to reinstate RUSADA as some government representatives perceived that the decision had been influenced by commercial interests in sport. In response via an open letter, Craig Reedie argued back:

> The accusation that WADA and me personally have pandered to the interests of money over clean sport are totally untrue, and deeply offensive. The author of those remarks, as a former Director General of WADA, should know better. This week's decision was based entirely on achieving Russian compliance, as properly delivered.
>
> (WADA, 2018b)

It is understandable that WADA, and Reedie in particular, refuted the allegation that they were conflicted. Yet, their language did not lend itself to reconciliation or the creation of viable working partnerships. Considering apologies can be perceived as a form of weakness, it is possible that any form of apology acknowledging wrongdoing from WADA in public statements would have presented further opportunities for organisations to challenge their legitimacy.

The refusal to admit negligence can also help explain WADA's focus on projecting success. A comparable conclusion can be drawn here with the work of Wagner and Pedersen (2014)43 who argued that the IOC promoted the success of its policy in an attempt to institutionalise its anti-doping campaign. In this case, while WADA disseminated a rhetoric of success, the tactics may have been enough to maintain legitimacy with more passive evaluators who were neither knowledgeable nor were actively assessing WADA. There are numerous examples of WADA's success rhetoric. For instance, WADA argued that the outcome of the first Pound Report was positive for anti-doping and clean athletes despite the scale of corruption involved (WADA, 48), thus reaffirming previous concerns that the biggest problem with anti-doping derives from a lack of stakeholder interest. The recommendations provided in the Pound Report exposed failings signifying to stakeholders that there were problems with the system. By presenting them as an opportunity, WADA created a narrative that the report was a success (WADA, 48). Following the publication of the second McLaren report, similar rhetoric was wielded by Reedie:

> The McLaren Investigation, and WADA's independent Commission that was led by Richard Pound in 2015, have successfully demonstrated the value of investigations – both as a regulatory tool and a key deterrent to doping. With the powers of investigation that were vested in WADA in the 2015 Code, the Agency became better equipped to protect clean athletes.
> (WADA, 2016b)

Despite the findings of both investigations undermining WADA's anti-doping system and the results of the 2014 Sochi Winter Olympics, the language and tone of Reedie's statement implied a victory for WADA. The focus on the success of the investigations and planned use of investigative methods for the future ignored that the testing system WADA had advocated since its inception was vulnerable to gross manipulation.

The rhetoric of winning and success was clear in responses to WADA's handling of RUSADA's reinstatement. After reinstating RUSADA, despite challenges from stakeholders, Reedie highlighted: 'We [WADA] have been able to declare compliant the Russian anti-doping agency because we have spent four years rebuilding it from the bad old days' (Doherty, 50), suggesting the decision was a victory for WADA. Similarly, when WADA finally retrieved the LIMS data from the Moscow laboratory, Reedie celebrated: 'By imposing those conditions, we now have gained access to the data and samples contained within the Moscow Laboratory that was, for so long, out of reach. It is currently being used to bring more cheats to justice with dozens of cases now proceeding through the various judicial channels' (Mackay, 51). The retrieval of data from the laboratory was a significant development for the ongoing investigation, however, there was no acknowledgement about the delay in retrieval. This positivity again reiterated an attempt to frame WADA's work as proactive, rather than reactive, to the biggest scandal of its existence. There was evidence of some contrition from WADA towards the end of Reedie's presidency as he admitted, 'What it [the scandal] taught us when it erupted was that we were not equipped to deal with such a large-scale program' (Grohmann, 52). The statement subtly implied that WADA was now better able to deal with this style of scandal.

WADA used specific rhetoric in response to legitimacy challenges in order to (1) present an image of control, (2) deny any wrongdoing and (3) reinterpret legitimacy challenges into WADA's successes. The benefit of using this language was that potential legitimacy challenges were presented as positive situations that minimised the opportunity for further criticism.

Conclusion

To conclude, this case has provided further insight into the legitimacy processes surrounding WADA during the biggest crisis of its existence. WADA was subject to legitimacy challenges from two different groups. The first group consisted of government representatives, athletes and NADOs, and the second group consisted of Olympic movement representatives. We demonstrated that the legitimacy challenges to WADA from the sport-governing bodies group were more threatening than the first group, because they suggested alternatives to WADA. In response to the challenges raised by the inter-governmental and sport-governing bodies groups, WADA's decisions were largely limited to reactive changes based upon limited reflection of the anti-doping system propagated under WADA and the IOC. The reactive approach was supported by rhetoric that positioned WADA as a successful, proactive organisation that denied any culpability. As the final chapter will develop in detail, WADA has displayed a pattern of defiant and manipulative behaviour in guarding its legitimacy. The consequences of this behavioural style for anti-doping, and the lessons available to other areas of governance, will now be discussed.

References

Altukhov, S., & Nauright, J. (2018). The new sporting Cold War: Implications of the Russian doping allegations for international relations and sport. *Sport in Society, 21*(8), 1120–1136.

Athletes failed by WADA decision to lift ban on Russian anti-doping agency. (2018). *The Australian*. Retrieved from https://www.theaustralian.com.au/.

Beacon, B. (2017, May 19). Athletes pushing for anti-doping charter of rights: WADA optimistic Russia will clean up abuses that have scandalized Olympics. *The Montreal Gazzette*. Retrieved from https://montrealgazzette.com/.

Butler, N. (2018, March 23). Exclusive: International Testing Agency head outlines conduct and independence of new body. Retrieved from https://www.insidethegames.biz.

Clarey, C. (2015, December 1). Cloud of corruption and doping hangs worldwide. *The New York Times*. Retrieved from https://www.nytimes.com/.

Dasgupta, L. (2017). Russian twister and the World Anti-Doping Code: Time to shun the elitist paradigm of anti-doping regime. *The International Sports Law Journal*, 17(1–2), 4–14.

Dickinson, M. (2015, November 10). Russia is laughing in the face of sporting justice. *The Times*. Retrieved from https://www.thetimes.co.uk/.

Doherty, C. (2018). Anti-doping boss says Russia on way to 'robust' system. Retrieved from Press Association via Nexis.com.

Gibson, O. (2015, November 11). A truly independent Wada should have the power to sanction sports and nations. *The Guardian*. Retrieved from www.theguardian.com/uk.

Gillespie, K. (2016, July 19). The Canadian who might get Russia kicked out of Rio. Toronto Star. Retrieved from https://www.thestar.com/.

Girginov, V., & Parry, J. (2018). Protecting or undermining the integrity of sport? The science and politics of the McLaren report. *International Journal of Sport Policy and Politics*, 10(2), 393–407.

Gleeson, M. (2018). IOC Athletes' Commission supports WADA's lifting of ban on RUSADA. *Reuters*. https://www.reuters.com/.

Grohmann, K. (2019). WADA was not equipped to handle size of Russian doping scandal -Reedie. *Reuters*. https://www.reuters.com/.

Hermann, A. (2019). The tip of the iceberg: The Russian doping scandal reveals a widespread doping problem. *Diagoras: International Academic Journal on Olympic Studies*, 3, 45–71.

Herman, M. (2016, July 18). Russian gymnasts must not be banned from Rio, says governing body. *Reuters*. Retrieved from https://uk.reuters.com/.

Hunt, T.M. (2011). *Drug games: The International Olympic Committee and the politics of doping, 1960–2008*. Austin, TX: University of Texas Press.

iNADO. (2015, November 16). iNADO urges action to protect clean sport. Retrieved from http://www.inado.org/about/press-releases.html.

iNADO. (2018b). NADO Leaders Group: International anti-doping leaders stand united with international athlete community in calling for meaningful reform of WADA governance. Retrieved from http://www.inado.org/press-releases.html.

iNADO. (2018a). NADO statement: iNADO dismayed at WADA compromise with Russia. Retrieved from http://www.inado.org/press-releases.html.

Ingle, S. (2016, July 23). Russia facing Olympic judgment day as IOC decides Rio 2016 fate. *The Guardian*. Retrieved from www.theguardian.com/uk.

Ingle, S. (2016, June 14). Athletes 'have lost faith' in IOC and Wada over Russia failures. *The Guardian*. Retrieved from www.theguardian.com/uk.

Ingle, S., & Gibson, O. (2016, September 21). IOC to set up anti-doping unit to curtail power of Wada. *The Irish Times*. Retrieved from https://www.irishtimes.com/.

IOC. (2017a). Joint statement following the meeting of IOC president, Prof. Richard Mclaren and WADA president. Retrieved from https://www.olympic.org/news/joint-statement-following-the-meeting-of-ioc-president-prof-richard-mclaren-and-wada-president.

IOC. (2017b). Independent testing authority on track. Retrieved from https://www.olympic.org/news/independent-testing-authority-on-track.

IOC. (2019). Statement from the IOC on WADA recommendations. *International Olympic Committee.* https://www.olympic.org/.

IOC promises to boost Wada's funding if it agrees to anti-doping reform. (2016, October 8). *The Guardian.* Retrieved from https://www.theguardian.com/sport/2016/oct/08/ioc-wada-funding-anti-doping-reform.

Kalinski, M.I. (2017). 'State-sponsored' doping: A transition from the former Soviet Union to present day Russia. *BLDE University Journal of Health Sciences, 2*(1), 1.

Lalovic, N. (2016, July 17). McLaren report weakened by leaked letter: WADA member. *Gulf Times.* Retrieved from https://www.gulf-times.com/.

LawInSport. (2016). CCES shares proposed reforms developed by 17 NADOs to strengthen and unify the global fight for clean sport. Retrieved from https://www.lawinsport.com/.

Mackay, D. (2019). WADA success since formation 20 years ago damaged by Russian doping scandal, admits Sir Craig. Retrieved from https://www.insidethegames.biz/.

Maese, R. (2019). Why WADA banned Russia from the Olympics and what it means. *The Washington Post.* https://www.washingtonpost.com/.

Majority of Russian athletes doping, alleges German documentary. (2014, December 5). CNN. Retrieved from https://edition.cnn.com/.

McLaren, R.H. (2016a) The Independent Person Report. Retrieved from https://www.wada-ama.org/.

McLaren, R.H. (2016b). The Independent Person 2nd Report. Retrieved from https://www.wada-ama.org/.

Pound, R.W., McLaren, R.H., & Younger, G. (2015). Independent Commission Report #1. Retrieved from https://www.wada-ama.org/en/resources/world-anti-doping-program/independent-commission-report-1.

Pound, R.W., McLaren, R.H., & Younger, G. (2016). Independent Commission Report #2. Retrieved from https://www.wada-ama.org/en/resources/world-anti-doping-program/independent-commission-report-2.

Report details Russian system to evade Olympic doping tests. (2016, May 14). New Delhi Times. Retrieved from https://www.newdelhitimes.com/.

Ruiz, R. (2016, August 1). Rare show of discord between I.O.C. and World Anti-Doping Agency over Russian scandal. *The New York Times.* Retrieved from https://www.nytimes.com/.

Russian state television will not broadcast Olympics without national team. (2016, December 5). Reuters. Retrieved from https://www.reuters.com/.

Savulescu, J. (2016, July 25). Should Russian athletes really be banned from competing in the Rio Olympics? Retrieved from https://theconversation.com/should-russian-athletes-really-be-banned-from-competing-in-the-rio-olympics-62962.

Slater, M. (2016, August 3). Russia defends right to compete but Wada blamed for scandal. *The Independent.* Retrieved from https://www.independent.co.uk/.

Tensions emerge at WADA meeting over Russia suspension. (2018, May 17). Sport 24. https://www.news24.com/.

'Triumph for money over clean sport': Ex-Wada head criticises Russia decision. (2018). *The Guardian*. https://www.theguardian.com/

Tygart, T.T. (2016, May 25). Come clean, Russia, or no Rio. *The New York Times*. Retrieved from https://www.nytimes.com/.

USADA. (2018). Statement on the WADA Executive Committee's decision to reinstate Russia from Travis T. Tygart, CEO, U.S. Anti-Doping Agency. USADA. https://www.usada.org/.

WADA. (2014). WADA announces details of Independent Commission. *World Anti-Doping Agency*. https://www.wada-ama.org/.

WADA. (2015). WADA welcomes Independent Commission's report into widespread doping in sport. *World Anti-Doping Agency*. https://www.wada-ama.org/.

WADA. (2016a). WADA to immediately probe new Russian doping allegations related to 2014 Sochi Olympics. *World Anti-Doping Agency*. https://www.wada-ama.org/.

WADA. (2016b). WADA Statement regarding conclusion of McLaren Investigation. *World Anti-Doping Agency*. https://www.wada-ama.org/.

WADA. (2018a). WADA Executive Committee decides to reinstate RUSADA subject to strict conditions. *World Anti-Doping Agency*. https://www.wada-ama.org/.

WADA. (2018b). An open letter on Russian anti-doping compliance from Sir Craig Reedie, President of the World Anti-Doping Agency. *World Anti-Doping Agency*. https://www.wada-ama.org/.

WADA in the crosshairs, as IOC members fume at late response. (2016, August 2). Channel NewsAsia. Retrieved from https://www.channelnewsasia.com/news/international.

Wagner, U., & Pedersen, K.M. (2014). The IOC and the doping issue—An institutional discursive approach to organizational identity construction. *Sport Management Review*, *17*(2), 160–173.

Waldie, P. (2016, June 20). WADA head defends action on doping, ties to IOC amid wave of criticism. *The Globe and Mail*. Retrieved from https://www.theglobeandmail.com/.

Walsh, D. (2015, November 8). Pariah state. *The Sunday Times*. Retrieved from https://www.thetimes.co.uk/.

Weston Phippen, J. (2016, July 28). The Olympics have always been political. *The Atlantic*. Retrieved from https://www.theatlantic.com/.

Wilson, S. (2016 November 16). WADA under attack again over Russian doping scandal. *The Associated Press*. Retrieved from https://apnews.com/.

Chapter 10

Managing the legitimacy of the World Anti-Doping Agency

This book began by highlighting that despite 20 years of anti-doping regulation under World Anti-Doping Agency (WADA), socially organised doping programs such as those exposed in the Russian Olympic doping scandal remained possible. Prompted by this starting position we have examined the progress WADA has made towards reaching its goal of doping-free sport. In doing so, we have discussed how a lack of behavioural support from signatories has limited the agency's effectiveness. Given the importance of behavioural support from stakeholders to the success of WADA, we used multi-level legitimacy theory to examine why organisations do or do not obtain behavioural support from stakeholders. This provided a basis from which we investigated the behavioural support WADA received from its stakeholders and constituents, to inform conclusions about its legitimacy. Drawing on evidence presented in the seven case studies, the final chapter summarises our findings in relation to the two guiding questions of the book: (1) how has WADA's legitimacy been challenged since its foundation and (2) how has WADA responded when its legitimacy has been challenged? In answer to the first question, we argue that the design and structure of the anti-doping system creates legitimacy challenges for WADA because there is a lack of consensus about the organisation's legitimacy. Consequently, WADA's authority to regulate anti-doping has been challenged by stakeholders with pragmatic interest, resources and financial independence to negate the fear of negative commercial or reputational repercussions, such as media sports and wealthy nations.

In response to the second question, the cases we have presented illustrate that WADA has responded to legitimacy challenges with defensive tactics, including defiance and manipulation in order to maintain the current Olympic philosophy (i.e., the spirit of sport) to anti-doping regulation. The problem with this pattern of response is that it limits the ability to consider alternative approaches while excluding stakeholders. Furthermore, how WADA perceived the value of a stakeholder's support was a significant factor in determining the organisation's response. Stakeholders that provided significant resources to WADA were more likely to receive a favourable response which influenced policy change. The chapter culminates in suggested reforms to WADA and anti-doping, informed by the key findings, to improve the progress of the organisation towards doping-free sport.

A house built on sand

The first finding refers to the contextual conditions surrounding the challenges to WADA's legitimacy. Drawing evidence from the seven case studies, we conclude that the establishment of WADA at the Lausanne Conference promoted the development of an anti-doping organisation influenced by the judgements and agendas of a select group of governments and the International Olympic Committee (IOC). WADA's creation and subsequent prominence were reinforced by the requirement for Olympic nations and sports to endorse the WADC as a stipulation of the Olympic Charter. From a theoretical perspective, the field of anti-doping has been characterised by institutional complexity as WADA has attempted to homogenise stakeholders from different backgrounds with varied resources, beliefs and objectives. Consequently, the field of anti-doping is characterised by a lack of consensus about WADA's legitimacy, especially during the periods following major crises. These judgements have been expressed as verbal or behavioural challenges when a stakeholder perceived that the potential risk of conforming to the behaviour outlined in the WADC (e.g., threatened core organisational objectives) was greater than the potential risk of financial or reputational damage following a challenge to WADA. This risk trade-off was influenced by a stakeholder's objectives (i.e., what could they gain from the challenge), independence (i.e., could they be coerced by WADA) and means (i.e., did they have the resources to challenge WADA). We will now develop the argument that WADA's legitimacy is hamstrung by a lack of consensus and discuss the implications.

Critical to understanding why WADA's legitimacy was weakly validated and has been subject to challenge throughout its existence is the theory of institutional complexity. To recap, institutional complexity (Greenwood, Raynard, Kodeih, Micelotta, & Lounsbury, 2011) proposes that organisations can exist in multiple fields, which subject them to multiple (sometimes contradictory) pressures (Friedland & Alford, 1991). When organisations grow and operate in multiple fields that are characterised by different pressures, leaders must decide how to navigate the conflicts. As demonstrated in chapter three, the establishment of WADA at the Lausanne Conference promoted the development of an anti-doping organisation informed by the judgements of a select group of governments. This group invested in WADA to ensure that sport maintained a clean image given its value to political, economic and social agendas, including national identification, brand value protection and population exercise levels. Along with the IOC's decision to compromise at Lausanne, the creation of WADA ensured that the spirit of sport and Olympism were privileged within anti-doping regulation to protect the image of sport. This combination of legitimacy judgements was imposed on WADA and focused on protecting the ideals of sport, which provided the platform for its current policy trajectory. Consequently, the expectations laid out in the WADC reflected this ideological commitment and placed considerable behavioural pressure on WADA signatories to conform.

We also observed that WADA's single-minded emphasis on the 'spirit of sport' was problematic because it conflicted with the athlete-centrism, politicisation and commercialisation logics. Firstly, *athlete-centrism* refers to beliefs that harm minimisation and athlete representation should be at the centre of anti-doping rather than policy idealism stemming from amateur ideals about the spirit of sport. The demand for WADA to treat recreational drugs separately to PEDs and obtain greater athlete involvement in policy is an example of this logic. Secondly, the *politicisation of sport* refers to how certain nations view sport as a part of a wider investment in soft power, as sporting success can boost the image and influence of a country (Grix & Carmichael, 2012). From this perspective, sporting performance is the priority rather than the spirit of sport, and appropriate behaviour is that which maximises performance. An example of this is the systematic doping witnessed in the Russian Olympic doping scandal designed to ensure Russian athletes were internationally successful. Finally, the *commercialisation of sport* logic captures how sport has been leveraged to generate large revenue streams for international federations, sponsors, broadcasters, teams and, to a lesser extent, athletes. From this position, an entertaining sporting spectacle that can be commercialised through the sale of broadcasting rights and sponsorships is the priority rather than the spirit of sport for public good. The protection of Lance Armstrong by the Union Cycliste Internationale (UCI), because of his marketability, is an example of the prioritisation of commercial logics.

Developing the idea that competing judgements based on different logics have been suppressed, institutional complexity can be categorised by logic compatibility, field prioritisation and jurisdictional overlap (Raynard, 2016). As noted, the behavioural expectations of anti-doping under the spirit of sport are not well matched (i.e., compatible) with athlete-centrism, politicisation or commercialisation. This incompatibility becomes absolute with the prioritisation of anti-doping and the spirit of sport in the Olympic Charter, which stipulates that all international federations and National Olympic Committees must be signatories to the WADC. This compliance mandate situation is what Raynard termed *restrained complexity*, as regardless of other internal organisational judgements and pressures, expected and therefore legitimate behaviour, is determined by the external prioritisation of anti-doping.

We have demonstrated through the case analyses that stakeholder judgements about WADA's legitimacy were suppressed through fear of negative financial or reputational repercussions and the expected gain of conforming with the dominant judgement. Individuals in the field of anti-doping render a judgement of propriety based on the logic (belief system) they prioritise. Therefore, jolts in the field of anti-doping offered an opportunity to promote a competing point of view to the opinion pronounced by WADA. However, the decision to express criticism or reject behavioural expectations was influenced by a risk-reward evaluation by stakeholders of complying with institutional pressures. A stakeholder's decision was affected by their objectives, independence and means. For example, in the whereabouts case, challenges were predominantly launched by organisations that were not dependent upon the IOC, such as the International Association of Football Federations (FIFA) and the International Tennis Federation (ITF). The organisations that challenged WADA's legitimacy had been financially successful operating their own anti-doping policies, and their internal logic of commercialisation was threatened by an increase in out-of-competition (OOC) testing facilitated by the whereabouts system.

Similarly, with the UCI, retrospective evidence, such as the Cycling Independent Reform Commission report (2015), revealed how the organisation protected Armstrong because of his commercial value. Again, this suppression created the conditions leading the UCI to challenge WADA's legitimacy. The International Federation of Professional Footballer's (FIFPro) negative comments about WADA's recreational drugs policy are an example of how athlete-centrism can clash with anti-doping policy, as the penalties for Guerrero were not consistent with popular assessments of fairness. Finally, the judgements expressed by international federations and certain WADA executives during the Russian doping scandal demonstrated suppressed beliefs about WADA's legitimacy by calling for change. Suppressed negative judgements were also recorded for individuals who held alternative perspectives about how anti-doping should be regulated and who advocated for other approaches.

The notion that WADA has created institutional pressures for signatories conveyed through the WADC has been identified in previous research (Girginov, 2006; Hanstad, 2008; Wagner, 2010, 2011). However, the consideration that WADA signatories exist under a state of restrained institutional complexity and seemingly consider the risk of expressing dissent has provided new insight into the legitimacy of WADA. Not only is WADA vulnerable to challenge due to a lack of consensus about WADA's role, policies and action, but the same line of reasoning can be extended to understand WADA's lack of effectiveness towards achieving its desired outcomes of harmonised anti-doping policy and creating doping-free sport (Houlihan & Hanstad, 2019).

In the absence of effective compliance monitoring mechanisms, signatories can engage with the WADC at a superficial level (Gray, 2019; Houlihan, 2014). Therefore, any improvements towards more effective anti-doping are minimised, as are unwanted impacts on political or commercial agendas. Wagner (2011) noted how FIFA avoided fully implementing the first edition of the WADC, while the actions of the UCI and Russian doping scandals are examples of superficial engagement. In these cases, we discussed how superficial compliance is not always deliberate. For example, in the case of some signatories, other pressures – such as financial austerity – potentially hindered the government funding allocation needed for rigorous anti-doping enforcement. Therefore, compliance issues may exist, but not because of deliberate subterfuge. Regardless of the motive for compliance issues, this situation highlights the need for better monitoring mechanisms as we will discuss in the final section of this chapter.

Resulting from our analysis, we suggest that the conditions under which WADA's legitimacy has been challenged can be attributed to the restrained institutional complexity WADA signatories are subject to, which stems from the outcomes of the Lausanne Conference and Olympic Charter. Subsequently, WADA has been challenged when stakeholders perceived that the level of incompatibility with their own agendas outweighed any benefits of conformity and/or the source possessed the requisite means and/or independence to express criticisms. This finding extends research into the development of anti-doping to explain WADA's lack of effectiveness (Houlihan & Hanstad, 2019). The low level of consensus concerning WADA's policies and its handling of jolts has led to a wide variety of legitimacy challenges, about which we will now draw some final observations and conclusions.

Limited scope for change

Turning our attention to how the WADA Executive Committee has responded to legitimacy challenges, the evidence presented in the preceding analysis demonstrated that the agency has predominantly relied on (1) defying and resisting criticism and (2) manipulating expectations of legitimate behaviour. The ubiquity of these two types of strategic response was shown to be linked to the type of legitimacy challenges that WADA faced. When confronted with challenges that scrutinised policy and organisation performance, the case evidence suggested that WADA Executive Committee members relied on various forms of manipulation. When WADA was faced with challenges to its moral and ideological reasoning (i.e., WADA's justification for its policies) and organisational purpose (i.e., WADA's responsibilities), the case evidence revealed that the agency relied on various forms of defiance. Both types of response illustrated that WADA's governors have been averse to accommodating concerns and critique. This finding is pertinent for anti-doping because the use of high agency strategies to avoid submission to legitimacy challenges means that external opinions are excluded from decision-making processes. Although acquiescence and compromise were not typical strategic responses, when WADA Committee members did compromise, we argue it was based on the perceived value of the challenger to the organisation.

To evaluate why WADA has engaged in high agency responses, we consider its decisions with respect to previous analyses of how organisations manage their legitimacy. It has been hypothesised that the likelihood of defiance and manipulation increases when (1) an organisation is subject to pressures from multiple stakeholders that (2) exhibit a lack of content consistency (Oliver, 1991). Content consistency refers to the degree of compatibility between challenger expectations and organisational goals. When organisations are expected to behave in a manner that differs from or hinders internal objectives, they are more likely to actively resist the pressures. Conversely, it has been theorised that organisations are less likely to resist challenges when they are dependent upon the support of a challenger for resources and survival, and the stakeholder has the means to coerce a response from an organisation (Black, 2008). This results in the prioritisation of certain stakeholders and their expectations, limiting an organisation's capacity for change. In the case of WADA, policy adaptation reflects the perspective of dominant field members.

Manipulating expectations of legitimate behaviour involves an organisation changing its role, purpose and activities through rhetoric and policy in order to retain authority, as opposed to trying to satisfy the demands of the audience (Oliver, 1991). In doing so, organisations can change the degree of consistency between the expectations of an evaluator and organisational behaviour. We have highlighted several instances of WADA responding to criticisms of their performance with manipulative strategies, of which the clearest example is the case of Lance Armstrong and the UCI. The actions of Armstrong highlighted how anti-doping tests could be beaten, and challenged the performance of WADA's testing system. If testing can be evaded throughout an athlete's career as with Armstrong, the legitimacy of WADA to regulate doping in sport, and protect athletes playing by the rules, is undermined. Consequently, WADA's Executive Committee responded with manipulation by influencing criteria for legitimate behaviour. Rather than directly addressing the issue of testing in their strategy and rhetoric, Executive Committee members construed the shortcomings of testing as a need for greater investigatory powers, extending the Executive Committee's reach as a regulatory organisation, and later reified in the 2015 WADC.

Manipulation was also evident in the success rhetoric discussed in relation to the Russian Olympic doping case. The exposure of systematic doping in Russia demonstrated the shortcomings of the WADA regime in detecting and regulating doping at a national level. Yet WADA's language throughout the incident consistently highlighted its positive actions and investigative successes, indicating an attempt to influence the content upon which its performance was judged (e.g., investigations, not testing). The final example of manipulation was provided in the whereabouts case study; however, it differed slightly as WADA utilised controlling manipulation over stakeholders who challenged the system. Multiple sport organisations questioned the practicalities of the whereabouts system due to the contexts of their sport (e.g., the ITF's concerns over the dynamic scheduling of professional tennis players). Manipulation via control is less subtle as organisations dictate new criteria for legitimate behaviour rather than influencing content upon which they are assessed. In the whereabouts system case, WADA threatened to remove each sport from the Olympic Games as a way of legitimating the system as a new activity that WADA should be responsible for. These examples demonstrate that when confronted with challenges based on inadequate performance, WADA has attempted to manipulate the criteria and content that it is judged against.

The second high agency response was WADA's defiance when faced with challenges about its moral reasoning and organisational purpose. Defiance differs from manipulation in that an organisation opposes challenges rather than reinterpreting them when consistency between challenges and organisational beliefs are low. There are multiple examples across cases that demonstrate this disregard for criticism. In relation to the whereabouts system, WADA consistently dismissed arguments that prioritised the human rights of athletes. WADA argued that the necessity of the whereabouts system for OOC testing was more important than an athlete's right to privacy in his or her personal life. The same line of reasoning was also observed with the TUE system. WADA adopted a dismissive approach by defying concerns over the potential misuse of therapeutic substances. The possibility that athletes should be entitled to medical treatment regardless of their occupation was considered inconsistent with concerns about substance misuse. The Armstrong case highlighted another example in the form of WADA's response to the UCI. Rather than just dismissing the challenges presented by the UCI, WADA actively sought to discredit the UCI's legitimacy. The key difference was that the arguments used to justify defiance focused on the source rather than the content of the criticism.

The finding that WADA has typically engaged in high agency responses has significant implications for anti-doping policy. The dominant use of defiance and manipulation suggests that the organisation is predisposed to implementing its own views through policies, and not listening to stakeholders when content consistency is low. Stiglitz (2003) demonstrated why high agency responses are problematic in regulatory organisations. Using the example of the International Monetary Fund, he noted that organisations become vulnerable to being captured by the internal interests of dominant members. Regulatory capture is feasible because the chain of accountability between those responsible for governing an international regulatory organisation and those affected by policy is frail. Therefore, it is very hard for those affected by decisions to voice concerns directly. The same process was observed in WADA's Executive Committee, which is primarily responsible for the direction of the organisation. The Committee draws membership from the Olympic movement and national government representatives, who were likely disinclined to review the current rationale for anti-doping and prohibition system given their desire to protect the image of sport.

The Executive Committee is overseen by the Foundation Board, again formed from the Olympic movement and national government representatives. The Foundation Board's structure reduces the accountability of the Executive Committee to the athletes impacted by policy, making defiance and manipulation to suit internal needs more viable. The World Health Organisation provides a similar example. The organisation was able to manipulate the meaning of external pressures by 'complying with reinterpreted demands' (Chorev, 2012, p. 92) so that policy remained a reflection of internal beliefs rather than external member views. If the processes within WADA do not ensure that the Executive Committee is held democratically accountable to those it protects (i.e., athletes), Executive Committee members may be more inclined to use high agency responses to protect internal interests.

The result of reinterpreting challenges to suit the internal beliefs of the organisation committee members is that it creates a limited scope in which policy adjustments can occur. Latitude for change is restricted to options that maintain internal organisational beliefs and the current Olympic philosophy approach to anti-doping regulation. WADA is flexible, but only within the confines of a narrow top-down prohibition frame. Therefore, policy development is at best incremental because anti-doping has a very limited scope for 'acceptable' change (e.g., governance practices, investigations, whistle-blower support) within the existing prohibition philosophy. These incremental changes give an appearance of flexibility without critical reconsideration of the rationales and aims of anti-doping. For example, we revealed WADA's reluctance to engage in fundamentally revising the recreational drugs policy. It has instead chosen to maintain a punitive approach in comparison to other drugs policies. WADA shows flexibility when it suits its philosophy but defies radical change when content consistency is low.

In addition to content consistency, stakeholder dependency is also relevant to understanding how WADA responded to behavioural and verbal challenges. Stakeholder dependency is the value that an organisation's leaders put on a positive evaluation of legitimacy from a stakeholder (Black, 2008). If an organisation relies on support (e.g., political lobbying or financial investment) from a stakeholder, it is more likely to meet the demands of criticism, regardless of content consistency. Equally, a regulatory organisation is more likely to comply with demands from stakeholders that have some form of power over the organisation (e.g., the ability to withdraw investment), or that cannot be coerced (e.g., are financially independent of the regulator). We argue that prioritisation of the IOC in anti-doping policy (as noted in chapter nine) is due to its position as the largest funder of WADA. WADA relies on this support and, therefore, the IOC has considerable power over the agency. Equally, WADA representatives were able to defy most stakeholders in relation to the whereabouts system but reached a compromise with FIFA. As one of the largest and most powerful international federations, FIFA did not fear Olympic expulsion and could not be coerced. Both examples highlight that the power relationships between anti-doping field members, and the ability to coerce or be coerced, have a significant bearing on legitimacy processes.

The treatment of athletes was another prominent example in the field of anti-doping that demonstrated the importance of coercion to institutional change. We argue that athletes have been ignored due to the fact that WADA does not materially depend on them for survival. For example, as discussed in chapter four, athletes went to the European Court of Human Rights to challenge WADA over the whereabouts system. Athletes recognised that they were more likely to see change if the challenge originated from a stakeholder to whom WADA was legally beholden. Similarly, WADA ignored information about Russian doping from athlete whistle-blowers, and it required an ARD documentary for WADA to acquiesce to calls for an investigation. Even WADA's decision to launch an investigation was determined, in part, by the public response. Our analysis suggests that WADA knew Russian doping would pose a serious challenge to its legitimacy and responding to the whistle-blowers with avoidance was unlikely to have negative repercussions. WADA's response to the Fancy Bear's data leak is another example of how stakeholder dependency influenced responses. The nations challenging WADA over the TUE system were those that had histories of doping and, apart from Russia, were not major Olympic nations. Their lack of perceived value to WADA may have made it easier to ignore them even if their criticisms were valid.

The policy approach adopted by WADA leads to two problems. The first problem with responding to stakeholders that issue challenges is that it typically involves a short-term approach and relegates consideration of fundamental changes in the rationale or approach that underpins the anti-doping system (Read, Skinner, Lock, & Houlihan, 2019). The short-term approach becomes more problematic when policies and responses are implemented that only aim to satisfy one stakeholder. An example is shown in our examination of the recreational drugs policy. It is apparent that the WADC was based on a need to satisfy the Olympic movement and select government representatives who did not want to tarnish the image of athletes as role models. WADA's focus on recreational drugs has since been criticised for being a waste of resources and outside of the organisation's remit (Waddington, Christiansen, Gleaves, Hoberman, & Møller, 2013). As the evidence suggested, if WADA continues to strategically respond to stakeholders dependent on their value to the organisation, it is unlikely that there will ever be a fundamental change in anti-doping policy.

The second problem with prioritising stakeholders is that it may disenfranchise stakeholders in the field of anti-doping who are continually defied and therefore become marginalised. Less powerful stakeholders may feel that they have no voice in determining rules and regulations, which may lead to a withdrawal of behavioural support. This is a significant issue when considering the growing demand from athletes for proper representation. If athlete judgements continue to be ignored, WADA risks losing further support from athlete bodies. The same argument pertains to NADOs who are represented by the NADO Advisory Group but have no formal representation at WADA despite being an integral part of anti-doping implementation. If the judgements of NADOs are marginalised, WADA again risks losing critical behavioural support. During the creation of WADA, the judgements of international federations and certain nations were ignored at the Lausanne Conference, as the conference was dominated by a few governments and powerful media sports. We suggest it is possible that the exclusion of the judgements held by marginalised organisations also contributed to the lack of behavioural support they later showed for anti-doping policy.

In summary, WADA has predominantly used high agency responses to challenges from a range of stakeholders. The significance of WADA's approach for anti-doping is that high agency responses in regulatory organisations exclude less powerful stakeholders from influencing policy. Given the lack of account-ability in WADA's governance structures and potentially conflicted committee members, WADA policy is highly vulnerable to regulatory capture. Regulatory capture means that the scope for change in anti-doping policy is limited to an internal view.

Legitimacy and accountability

Considered together, the two previous sections highlight why legitimacy, de-fined as 'the perceived appropriateness of an organization to a social system in terms of rules, values, norms, and definitions' (Deephouse, Bundy, Tost, & Suchman, 2017, p. 32), will always be a problem for WADA, and anti-doping generally, due to its lack of formal accountability. The design of WADA's governance system and regime entrenched institutional complexity into the anti-doping system. As a result, the governance system has always been squeezed between the pressures imposed through the WADC and the objectives of commercial and national sports groups. WADA imposes anti-doping policies, justified through claims about protecting the spirit of sport and deployed through a global regime relying upon a diverse selection of sport organisations and countries with their own values. It has been a collision of competing agendas that was inevitably going to create problems for behavioural support and compliance. Arguably, it has only been through coercion wherein the IOC has mandated compliance with the WADC that WADA attracted signatories and bound them to a narrow ideological and regulatory commitment. WADA's legitimacy therefore remains in a state of weak validity as it is not grounded in a commonly shared judgement of propriety between evaluators (i.e., low con-sensus between members) as demonstrated by the challenges it has faced and the lack of support it has received. The cases examined in this book brought these severe challenges to the surface and cast doubt upon WADA's future without a strong platform for its anti-doping policy legitimacy.

Our analysis of WADA's responses to legitimacy challenges suggested that the organisation's leaders have undermined the behavioural support they sought and demanded from stakeholders. We found that WADA has not typically engaged with evaluators when they have expressed challenges. Legitimacy challenges represented an expression from stakeholders that WADA was not perceived to meet its propriety judgement of appropriate behaviour.

WADA's dependence on high agency strategies to resist legitimacy challenges and prioritisation of stakeholders based on their perceived value to the organisation necessarily excluded other major field members such as athletes and NADOs. WADA's response has been compounded by its own governance structure which allows the Executive Committee to create policy aligned with its internal beliefs, in turn constraining the organisation's capability to change. These internal beliefs appear to prioritise stakeholders and other key organisations that WADA perceived to be most valuable or influential. The outcome for WADA has been that the weak validity that it was founded upon has not improved, with survival still dependent on the legitimacy support of a handful of powerful stakeholders. We argue that the relationship between restrained institutional complexity, high agency responses, legitimacy and effectiveness can be connected by inspecting the organisation's accountability.

Given the diversity of stakeholders, WADA is beholden to, responding in a way that satisfies the expectations of all parties is not feasible. Therefore, WADA cannot be accountable to the demands of all stakeholders, all the time, which undermines the organisation's legitimacy when conceptualised as a collective consensus between field members. Proposed by Koppell (2005), 'multiple accountabilities disorder' theorises the problem regulatory organisations face when working in environments characterised by a plurality of stakeholder beliefs and consequently try to satisfy multiple, competing expectations of accountability. Organisations become stymied by trying to balance constituent involvement in regulatory processes and organisational effectiveness (Schillemans & Bovens, 2011). Koppell differentiated five elements of accountability: liability, transparency, controllability, responsibility and responsiveness. Accordingly, expectations of accountability may refer to whether (1) an organisation can be reprimanded for poor performance, (2) internal decision-making processes are shared publicly, (3) the expectations of controlling bodies (e.g., the foundation board) are met, (4) the organisation follows its own rules and (5) the expectations of stakeholders are met. If an organisation attempts to simultaneously satisfy all these versions of accountability, it is likely to perform poorly because of conflicting behavioural expectations (Balboa, 2017). For instance, in being responsive to one stakeholder's concern, an organisation may violate socially expected standards of behaviour, leading to a state of organisational limbo where no group is satisfied. Organisations that cannot balance accountability demands risk losing legitimacy, and therefore behavioural support (Black, 2008).

WADA certainly operates in a field characterised by complexity, and where being responsive to all constituent challenges is virtually impossible. Koppell (2005) observed: 'No organization can be consistently responsive to a diverse set of interests. There is generally no agreed-upon hierarchy of the needs of any given community' (p. 104). In responding to complex fields, regulatory organisations face the problem of suffering the opposite of multiple accountabilities disorder – single accountability disorder (Balboa, 2017). Single accountability disorder describes an organisational state where senior leaders pursue a single objective to which they are accountable in order to survive, ignoring other constituent demands. Advocates of single accountability disorder argue that an organisation would never achieve anything if it tried to balance all constituent demands within a single strategy (Balboa, 2017). However, it is possible that the single accountabilities approach can be productive until pressure increases from excluded stakeholders (e.g., threatening to withdraw financial support). This appears to be the case with WADA, an organisation that has prioritised accountability to its core funders, displacing other constituent demands. Therefore, WADA's vulnerability to legitimacy challenges stems from an accountability ambiguity between pressure to prioritise the IOC for survival (single accountability) and expectations to represent all stakeholder demands (multiple accountabilities). As long as the Executive Committee cannot satisfy the demands of every stakeholder, WADA's legitimacy will remain trapped between single and multiple accountability disorders and be challenged.

WADA must inevitably seek to balance its accountability imperatives in order to retain legitimacy, namely, liability, transparency, controllability, responsibility and responsiveness. Balancing accountability involves promoting collaboration and participation between stakeholders rather than responding to all demands. Therefore, constituents can be valued in other ways, such as having a meaningful input into policy forums supported by adequate transparency to provide information on organisational performance (Schillemans, 2015). In making changes to balance aspects of accountability, we argue that WADA should, in theory, increase legitimacy with stakeholders who want to improve anti-doping efforts. Yet, if organisations that prioritise commercial and nationalist objectives perceive that they no longer gain utility from WADA, the organisation risks provoking a powerful stakeholder group and being exposed to further legitimacy challenges. This contradiction exemplifies why WADA's task is so complex, as they find themselves competing with a complex web of social, political and commercial interests. Accountability deficits create a further problem in terms of legitimacy. To counter stakeholders that privately do not support anti-doping, the primary solution would be to give WADA greater responsibility to monitor, investigate and sanction compliance issues. However, there may be little political support within anti-doping to give WADA this level of responsibility. Therefore, in addition to increased monitoring and sanctioning powers, greater liability, transparency and control would be required by the Executive Committee and Foundation Board to ensure that the powers were implemented transparently and equally.

A multifaceted assessment of WADA's legitimacy helps fulfil this book's aim of analysing the legitimacy of WADA from a multi-level perspective and to identify why there is a lack of behavioural support that is inhibiting WADA's effectiveness. Due to the nature of its global task and the varied stakeholders in the field of anti-doping, WADA is unlikely to achieve strong legitimacy, defined as the widespread consensus of positive judgements. The lack of behavioural support undermining the effectiveness of WADA can be explained in part as a consequence of the private, negative propriety judgements held by some stakeholders due to political, social and commercial conflicts of interest. This situation has been compounded by the make-up of the Executive Committee, which comprises the Olympic movement and government representatives who are both vulnerable to conflicting interests and competing accountabilities. If WADA does not engage in reform, the effectiveness of anti-doping will always be limited as it will struggle to convince stakeholders to support them. The following section examines the governance changes WADA has introduced since 2018 and offers direction for further areas for reform.

Reforming WADA

It is easy to criticise anti-doping efforts without offering feasible changes to help reinforce the agency's legitimacy and effectiveness. The final part of this chapter provides structural and governance recommendations to improve WADA's performance. We argue that the issues highlighted in this chapter can be addressed by targeting WADC implementation structures and governing activities. Recommendations are presented that aim to minimise complexity. These recommendations focus on two areas: (1) the current structures through which anti-doping policy is implemented and (2) developing mechanisms to improve the transparency of governing activities. By embedding democratic methods in governing activities, placing internal accountability on officials to follow rules and ensuring responsibility to all constituents, it is possible to address WADA's weak legitimacy.

Improving WADA's perceived legitimacy via governance and structural reform should also improve the effectiveness of the organisation as a regulatory body and reduce the likelihood of unethical behaviour (Geeraert, 2018). Our analysis has demonstrated, if WADA were to be abolished, sport's diverse constituents are unlikely to ever reach an agreement about how anti-doping should be managed. Moreover, it is doubtful that sports organisations would give up as much control as they ceded in 1999 at Lausanne, forcing a return to the situation that preceded WADA where sport organisations were self-regulating without oversight. Despite current shortcomings, we conclude that it would be more productive to reform WADA into an organisation capable of effectively regulating drugs in sport, than it would be to disband the agency and attempt to create a new regulatory institution.

The first issue to be addressed is the institutional complexity within which signatories exist. A significant source of challenges to WADA's legitimacy has been from signatories that are seemingly unconcerned with anti-doping, or who have prioritised other issues. Consequently, a system that reduces this conflict should improve the effectiveness of the organisation. To respond to signatories who do not prioritise anti-doping, structural change should be made to increase the independence of policy implementation and organisational responsibility for doping. By increasing independence and responsibility, signatories operating under conflicting pressures have less opportunity to subvert anti-doping policy and will bear greater responsibility for the implications with disregarding anti-doping efforts.

Before suggesting specific reforms, we caution that any structural changes to policy implementation are given on the assumption that WADA's governance would also be developed to ensure stakeholders are adequately represented in decision-making, and that WADA's management boards are held accountable for their actions by a wider range of stakeholders. WADA has recently supported changes in policy implementation and compliance monitoring to address conflicted stakeholders that are worth outlining. The foundation of the ITA in 2018 as an organisation to take over testing implementation for international federations and sports events organisers is a positive step towards dealing with institutional complexity. Organisations that work with the ITA relinquish responsibility for managing anti-doping, reducing the capacity for interference. However, the ITA has been previously criticised for lacking independence from the IOC (Butler, 2018). Therefore, in addition to the ITA, WADA's continued focus on improving its investigatory capacity and supporting whistle-blowers is another way of deterring non-compliance. WADA's ISO9001:2015 Code Compliance Monitoring Program and 2019 Compliance Strategy, are also constructive developments towards ensuring signatories fully implement the code. The Compliance Strategy provides the ability to audit signatories, while the continuous monitoring of signatory activities helps WADA move away from simple quantitative methods of assessment (e.g., how many tests conducted per year). Consistency between in-depth monitoring of signatories will be crucial to certify equality of treatment but will require significant funds to ensure parity between parties targeted.

The ITA and Code Compliance Monitoring Program should lead to increases in stakeholder's perceptions of WADA's legitimacy, especially to stakeholders who prioritise anti-doping. It will also likely persuade conflicted organisations to comply with the WADC. Previously, WADA lacked the capacity to sanction signatories for non-compliance. The introduction of the International Standard for Code Compliance by Signatories (ISCCS), to allow WADA to impose varying levels of sanctions on non-compliant signatories, adds further weight to the coercive pressure available to WADA. This coercion must also be accompanied by technical and material resource provision to ensure that local sport anti-doping programmes, which are unable to comply or inadvertently non-complying, are not treated in the same manner as signatories who choose not to comply.

The ITA, ISCCS and Code Compliance Monitoring Program will all contribute to ensuring that the anti-doping system will be implemented more equitably, however, these changes do not ensure that policy is implemented substantively. We argue that to ensure the implementation of the WADC progresses from a superficial level (i.e., policy implementation to avoid non-compliance) to committed action (i.e., policy implementation to reduce doping), signatories must bear greater responsibility for the actions of athletes under their remit. At present, signatories are responsible only for implementation, not the effectiveness of anti-doping activities. A chain of responsibility that connects the behaviour of athletes to consequences for other major stakeholders including managers, team owners, national sporting bodies, international federations and Olympic Committees could incentivise these stakeholders to seriously engage in the prevention and monitoring of their athletes. If sport organisations were to face economic and reputational consequences for the actions of their athletes, there would be an added incentive to prevent doping and educate athletes. The International Weightlifting Federation (IWF) has set a precedent for this model as member federations can receive sanctions such as the loss of financial support, fines and suspension from IWF events for up to four years, if one or more of their athletes or an affiliated individual (e.g., coach) commits an anti-doping rule violation. This does raise questions about collective responsibility if a member federation were to be banned from events, effectively banning athletes who have not committed any rule violations. However, a graded sanction system starting with economic penalties and progressing in severity may offer a solution.

The problem that arises with a chain of responsibility is the potential for signatories to cover up doping to avoid the consequences of public censure. The case of Lance Armstrong provided an example of how sports organisations may conceal doping for commercial reasons. As a result, independence and monitoring become critical. If testing, results management and sanctioning were all managed by independent entities, such as the ITA, there would be less chance for interference in case management. Likewise, enhanced code compliance monitoring should help identify and address compliance issues. The notion of a chain of responsibility with increased independence is not proposed to give WADA further powers to coerce compliance, but to address the inherent complexity in the field of anti-doping that undermines its legitimacy and makes its mandate so complex and contradictory. As previously noted, if anti-doping implementation were to be further separated from conflicted organisations, any increases in WADA's capacities would need to be accompanied by improved governance to ensure that new powers are implemented fairly and that all stakeholders are represented in policy design.

The second structural recommendation is for WADA to investigate alternative funding models that reduce its dependency on the Olympic movement. In 2018, WADA's Foundation Board agreed to an annual 8% budget increase for four years (WADA, 2018a). However, this modest escalation in budget size does not reduce WADA's dependence on the IOC as a 50% contributor. Furthermore, WADA's expected budget for 2020 of US$38,974,738 ($18,722,369 from public authorities matched by the IOC, plus an additional $1,530,000 from Montreal International) would not even earn them a place in the current top 25 highest-earning athletes list (Forbes, 2020), and suggests that budget constraints are due to a lack of priority rather than a lack of resources. Sponsorship and broadcasting rights are a significant income stream within sport, and direct contributions or a percentage levy on these revenue sources may ease WADA's reliance on the IOC. Bańka highlighted that if WADA is to be more effective, it must find new sources of funding, possibly through sponsors (Mackay, 2019). As with any financial change, WADA will need to ensure that it does not become conflicted between new financial sources, adding to its accountability ambiguities. For example, a levy on sponsors and broadcasters could create new stakeholders to whom WADA is accountable. In addition, a levy may create a situation where the agency's survival is dependent on sport's ability to attract sponsorship. Additionally, increasing the number of contributors may further reduce the influence of poorer nations who financially contribute little. Although a restructured financial model has the potential to improve WADA's legitimacy, it must not worsen the same problem of dependence as the current configuration and transfer power to a select few sponsors that want to maintain the high performance at all costs nature of sport.

Before providing governance recommendations, it should be noted that since 2016, WADA has been in the process of reforming its governance structures and policies. In November 2016, WADA's Foundation Board approved the formation of a Governance Working Group to evaluate the policies and structures of the organisation's decision-making bodies (WADA, 2016). Two years later, in November 2018, WADA's Foundation Board approved a further series of specific recommendations put forward by the Governance Working Group including:

- Ensuring the President and Vice-President are independent.
- Two new independent seats with voting rights on the Executive Committee.
- A nominations committee to vet potential committee members.
- A nine-year limit on membership with the WADA Executive Committee, Foundation Board and standing committees.
- Formation of an ethics board to oversee Executive Committee behaviour.
- One seat on all WADA standing committees for athlete and NADOs representatives (WADA, 2018b).

We argue that these changes suggest a willingness to make some compromises in order to meet legitimacy challenges, as WADA President Sir Craig Reedie suggested, 'The review of WADA's governance model has been comprehensive and has clearly shown WADA's willingness to adapt' (WADA, 2018b). Furthermore, at the WADA symposium in March 2019, Reedie indicated that in the future an athlete representative with voting rights could sit on the Executive Committee (Brown, 2019) to represent athletes. The burden, however, remains on athletes to establish a mechanism for deciding how they would elect such an individual; a task complicated by the diversity of athletes across sport and nations. Under new WADA President Witold Bańka, the organisation's strategic plan for 2020–2024 includes being athlete-centred as a priority.

The question remains, to what extent do WADA's proposed changes deal with institutional complexity, improve vulnerability to regulatory capture, reduce prioritisation and manage accountability. The first governance working group recommendation that all new WADA Presidents and Vice-Presidents are independent was a significant step towards reducing the chance of regulatory capture. Previous WADA Presidents and Vice-Presidents have been active serving members of the Olympic movement and national governments. Dual roles meant that they were more vulnerable to conflicts of interest, potentially squeezed between doing what is best for anti-doping and what is in the best interests of the other entity they represent. In theory, the election of a new WADA President and Vice-President who does not hold any responsibility to a government or sporting institution reduces the likelihood that WADA decision-making will be vulnerable to regulatory capture. However, new WADA President Witold Bańka is a former Polish politician and national sprinter, and his relationship with these two significant stakeholders is yet to be tested in the manner the Russian Olympic doping scandal tested Sir Craig Reedie. The addition of two independent Executive Committee members with voting rights and an independent nominations committee should also help reduce the chance of regulatory capture and stakeholder prioritisation by introducing competing opinions at an executive level. The nine-year limit on membership with the WADA Executive Committee, Foundation Board and standing committees will also improve the democratic turnover of governors to avoid regulatory capture.

The creation of a nominations committee to vet potential committee members will provide a helpful safeguard to ensure that individuals with appropriate skills and independence are chosen rather than individuals with vested interests. These changes to improve independence are positive, but do not fully address the propensity of WADA's Executive Committee to prioritise legitimacy sources. More independent members would dilute the concentration of conflicted representatives on the committee. The ongoing formation of an ethics board to oversee adherence to a code of ethical behaviour (at the time of writing this book was currently being formalised) is important for accountability, and for ensuring that all committee members behave in a manner consistent with expectations. However, without knowing what rules will be presented in the code of ethics, it is hard to determine the utility of this reform.

The last reform, provision of one seat on all WADA standing committees for athlete and NADOs representatives (WADA, 2018b) does promote competing judgements in governance processes, however, without voting rights there is no change in democratic representation. Upon inspection, the reforms proposed by the Governance Working Group are positive steps for the administration of anti-doping, but the fundamental issues we have identified in relation to legitimacy and accountability remain. In response, we provide several additional suggestions to improve the effectiveness of WADA that address regulatory capture, stakeholder prioritisation and accountability resulting from the high agency strategies.

Recommendations

The first recommendation to prevent capture and prioritisation is to reform eligibility criteria for the Executive Committee. In theory, if the Committee were staffed by experienced and informed individuals who were all independent from the Olympic movement and government positions, the chance of regulatory capture and prioritisation would be significantly reduced. However, it is unlikely that these two stakeholders would rescind control in this manner and allow independent individuals to determine how they should be regulated. Therefore, it may be more feasible to reconsider how the Foundation Board functions as an oversight mechanism. High agency responses were possible due to the lack of direct accountability on the Executive Committee to field members. If the Executive Committee makes decisions that benefit the committee's dominant members, then the 38-member Foundation Board should provide oversight on these actions and decisions to stop prioritisation. Like the Executive Committee, the Foundation Board is conflicted by the equal split of Olympic movement members and government representatives. Consequently, there is a lack of adequate oversight as the Foundation Board is equally vulnerable to prioritisation and regulatory capture.

There are several options related to the lack of oversight that may change the perceived legitimacy of WADA and improve behavioural support from signatories. Firstly, independent positions with full voting rights could be created in the Foundation Board, like those for the Executive Committee, in order to improve accountability. Secondly, to improve representation, a greater diversity of stakeholders integral to anti-doping could be included, such as athletes, NADOs and academics who are currently limited to standing committees. A more drastic approach would involve the remodelling of the Foundation Board so that it was composed of a representative from each sport and nation elected by athletes, officials and members. Finally, collective bargaining between athlete unions such as the World Players Association and WADA's Executive Committee could foster better representation and accountability. If an international athlete union was able to adequately represent the needs of all athletes subject to WADA's conditions, they could petition the agency in order to influence policy decisions. This mechanism is arguably more justifiable from a democratic standpoint than stricter policies determined by international federations, government representatives and WADA, because the rules would be at least partially determined by the individuals subject to them. It is known that the punishments for doping can be less severe in collectively bargained systems, such as the National Football League in the United States. However, policies that are collectively bargained tend to be based on a health perspective that privileges athlete well-being. Such policies discourage doping, not because it is morally wrong, but because it is potentially detrimental to long-term athlete health.

The previous structural and governance recommendations are admittedly broad and made with an appreciation that it took exposure of systematic doping in Russia for WADA to implement change. The evidence we have presented suggests that rather than waiting for another scandal or jolt to challenge its legitimacy, those looking to reform WADA (e.g., athlete groups) should aim to partner with powerful organisations that can leverage their authority over the organisation. The current omission of sponsors' and broadcasters' contributions to anti-doping is one potential group that could be convinced to exert pressure on the sports movement, and consequently WADA, to bolster anti-doping effectiveness. The threat of losing sponsor and broadcaster income may be sufficient to pressure conflicted signatories and WADA members to pursue anti-doping more actively.

In summary, the structural reforms we have presented to increase independence and mitigate against institutional complexity would ease the challenge WADA faces in regulating such a complex network of stakeholders and address the lack of behavioural support identified. WADA, however, as a regulatory organisation would also need to engage in significant governance reform. Without changes to the current organisational design that creates vulnerability to regulatory capture, enables stakeholder prioritisation and lacks accountability, any structural changes may be symbolic and continue to allow WADA to respond through defiance to continued legitimacy challenges.

Conclusion

The aim of this book was to explore the relationship between the legitimacy of WADA and its stakeholders. To guide this aim, two central questions were pursued:

1. How has WADA's legitimacy been challenged since its foundation?
2. How has WADA responded when its legitimacy has been challenged?

The insights presented in this final chapter have drawn together the analyses from the seven cases to elucidate the relationship between the legitimacy of WADA and its stakeholders. In short, WADA's legitimacy is always going to be vulnerable to challenge because of the diverse array of stakeholders – with competing priorities – it must satisfy. The lack of behavioural support that contributes to WADA's ineffectiveness is explained by the lack of consensus and suppressed negative judgements of its legitimacy. The suppression of deviant judgements about the legitimacy of anti-doping provides a constant source of tension. The complexity arises from the way WADA was formed at the Lausanne Conference. This created a hybrid system that prioritised select governments and the IOC. The hybrid design has since been problematic for

WADA, as responses to behavioural challenges have been guided by the principle of the 'spirit of sport' and organisational survival. Consequently, alternative views and approaches have been largely excluded from anti-doping policy reform. Without significant governance reform, it is likely that WADA will continue to respond in the same manner and will perpetually struggle to develop consensus between stakeholders to achieve its stated goal of doping free-sport.

Recognising the problems that arise from the current design of the anti-doping system, if it is to be effective with the widespread active support from athletes and anti-doping signatories that deters and detects doping, nuanced reform is required. Ensuring that policy is implemented rigorously and independently is the first step towards addressing the complexity of elite sport. Structural changes to the anti-doping system must be accompanied by governance reform to confirm that the risk of stakeholder prioritisation and regulatory capture are minimised. Although our analysis has demonstrated the vulnerability of WADA's legitimacy to being challenged, the agency remains the most viable option to achieve doping-free sport. This is because its ineffectiveness serves those who may not prioritise anti-doping, whilst simultaneously offering the only realistic opportunity for progress to groups who do prioritise anti-doping. By appreciating that legitimacy at a macro-level can vary in terms of the underlying consensus, WADA represents the apparent paradox of an organisation being both legitimate and constantly vulnerable to challenge.

The insight we have provided into WADA's legitimacy provides clarity about the tasks other global regulatory organisations within sport, and in society at large, face in achieving committed behavioural support. Transnational organisations like WADA will never be able to adequately satisfy the expectations of legitimate behaviour from all stakeholders to which they are beholden. Yet, they can endeavour to create a regulatory system that is sufficiently independent in implementation to minimise interference, whilst adopting a governance model that enables satisfactory accountability and responsibility to empower stakeholder engagement without risk of prioritisation or regulatory capture. Striking this balance in the highly politicised and commercialised world of elite sport presents a significant and ongoing challenge for WADA.

References

Balboa, C.M. (2017). Mission interference: How competition confounds accountability for environmental nongovernmental organizations. *Review of Policy Research, 34*(1), 110–131.

Black, J. (2008). Constructing and contesting legitimacy and accountability in polycentric regulatory regimes. *Regulation & Governance, 2*(2), 137–164.

Brown, A. (2019). WADA Symposium Day 1: Anti-doping gets more complicated as WADA evolves. *The Sports Integrity Initiative*. Retrieved from https://www.

sportsintegrityinitiative.com/wada-symposium-day-1-anti-doping-gets-more-complicated-as-wada-evolves/.

Butler, N. (2018). *Exclusive: International Testing Agency head outlines conduct and independence of new body.* Retrieved from https://www.insidethegames.biz/articles/1063026/exclusive-international-testing-agency-head-outlines-conduct-and-independence-of-new-body.

Chorev, N. (2012). 'A new health order as part of the new social order': The strategic response of the WHO to its member states. In *Political Power and Social Theory* (pp. 65–100). Emerald Group Publishing Limited.

Cycling Independent Reform Commission. (2015). Report to the president of the Union Cycliste Internationale. Cycling Independent Reform Commission. Lausanne, Switzerland.

Deephouse, D.L., Bundy, J., Tost, L.P., and Suchman, M.C., 2017. Organizational legitimacy: Six key questions. In Greenwood, R., et al. (Eds.), *The SAGE handbook of organizational institutionalism* (2nd ed., p. 223). Thousand Oaks, CA: Sage.

Forbes. (2020). The world's highest paid athletes 2020. Retrieved from https://www.forbes.com/.

Friedland, R., & Alford, R.R. (1991). Bringing society back in: Symbols, practices and institutional contradictions. In W.W. Powell & P.J. DiMaggio (Eds.), *The New Institutionalism in Organizational Analysis* (pp. 232–267). Chicago, IL: University of Chicago Press.

Geeraert, A. (2018). *National Sports Governance Observer. Final report.* Play the Game/Danish Institute for Sports Studies.

Girginov, V. (2006). Creating a corporate anti-doping culture: The role of Bulgarian sports governing bodies. *Sport in Society, 9*(2), 252–268.

Gray, S. (2019). Achieving compliance with the World Anti-Doping Code: Learning from the implementation of another international agreement. *International Journal of Sport Policy and Politics, 11*(2), 247–260.

Greenwood, R., Raynard, M., Kodeih, F., Micelotta, E.R., & Lounsbury, M. (2011). Institutional complexity and organizational responses. *The Academy of Management Annals, 5*(1), 317–371.

Grix, J., & Carmichael, F. (2012). Why do governments invest in elite sport? A polemic. *International Journal of Sport Policy and Politics, 4*(1), 73–90.

Hanstad, D.V. (2008). Drug scandal and organizational change within the International Ski Federation: A figurational approach. *European Sport Management Quarterly, 8*(4), 379–398.

Houlihan, B. (2014). Achieving compliance in international anti-doping policy: An analysis of the 2009 World Anti-Doping Code. *Sport Management Review, 17*(3), 265–276.

Houlihan, B., & Hanstad, D. V. (2019). The effectiveness of the World Anti-Doping Agency: Developing a framework for analysis. *International Journal of Sport Policy and Politics, 11*(2), 203–217.

Koppell, J.G. (2005). Pathologies of accountability: ICANN and the challenge of 'multiple accountabilities disorder'. *Public Administration Review, 65*(1), 94–108.

Mackay, D. (2019). Bańka to urge sponsors to back WADA in anti-doping battle. Inside The Games. https://www.insidethegames.biz/.

Oliver, C. (1991). Strategic responses to institutional processes. *Academy of Management Review*, 16(1), 145–179.

Raynard, M. (2016). Deconstructing complexity: Configurations of institutional complexity and structural hybridity. *Strategic Organization*, 14(4), 310–335.

Read, D., Skinner, J., Lock, D., & Houlihan, B. (2019). Legitimacy driven change at the world anti-doping agency. *International Journal of Sport Policy and Politics*, 11(2), 233–245.

Schillemans, T. (2015). Managing public accountability: How public managers manage public accountability. *International Journal of Public Administration*, 38(6), 433–441.

Schillemans, T., & Bovens, M. (2011). The challenge of multiple accountability. In Dubnick M. J. & Frederickson H. G. (Eds.), *Accountable governance: Problems and promises*. Armonk, NY: M. E. Sharpe.

Stiglitz, J.E. (2003). Democratizing the International Monetary Fund and the World Bank: Governance and accountability. *Governance*, 16(1), 111–139.

WADA. (2016). WADA Executive Committee and Foundation Board meetings. Retrieved from https://www.wada-ama.org/sites/default/files/resources/files/summary_notes_-_ec_fb_meeting_-november_2016.pdf.

WADA. (2018a). WADA Foundation Board endorses budget increase to strengthen agency's capacity to deliver clean sport.

WADA. (2018b). WADA Foundation Board approves wide-ranging governance reform. Retrieved from https://www.wada-ama.org/en/media/news/2018-11/wada-foundation-board-approves-wide-ranging-governance-reform.

Waddington, I., Christiansen, A.V., Gleaves, J., Hoberman, J., & Møller, V. (2013). Recreational drug use and sport: Time for a WADA rethink? *Performance Enhancement & Health*, 2(2), 41–47.

Wagner, U. (2010). The international cycling union under siege—Anti-doping and the biological passport as a mission impossible? *European Sport Management Quarterly*, 10(3), 321–342.

Wagner, U. (2011). Towards the construction of the world anti-doping agency: Analyzing the approaches of FIFA and the IAAF to doping in sport. *European Sport Management Quarterly*, 11(5), 445–470.

Appendix A

Events that have put WADA in the news

Date	News Stories
July 1999 to	Sydney Summit
December 1999	The Independence of WADA questioned
January 2000 to June 2000	Anticipation of WADA's first meeting
July 2000 to	USA Track and Field allows WADA to do testing
December 2000	ADRVs at Sydney Olympics
	EU works with WADA
January 2001 to June 2001	Lahti scandal
July 2001 to	Montreal selected for WADA headquarters
December 2001	FIFA resists WADA
	Gene doping emerges
January 2002 to June 2002	Testing for Salt Lake City Olympics
	IF/EU argument over funding
	First WADC draft
July 2002 to	UCI conflict with WADA, and Hein Verbruggen
December 2002	quits WADA
January 2003 to June 2003	Shane Warne ADRV
	IFs resisting WADC
	WADA not receiving payments from signatories
July 2003 to	Shane Warne ADRV
December 2003	IFs resisting WADC
	UCI and Pound argument over leaked Tour de France report
	Bay Area Laboratory Co-Operative (BALCO) scandal
January 2004 to June 2004	Greg Rusedski AAF
	BALCO scandal continues
	Dwayne Chamber and Marion Jones ADRV
July 2004 to	UCI conflict about handling of Tour de France report
December 2004	Negative report from WADA about Association of Tennis Professionals
	Marion Jones ADRV
	Dick Pound's independence as WADA President criticised

(Continued)

Date	News Stories
January 2005 to June 2005	Designer steroids and Major League Baseball
	Canadian customs confiscate new designer steroid
	Turin Games used to get governments to sign WADC
	WADA funding issues
	Caffeine prohibition
	Australian Football League refuses to sign WADC
	Nandrolone tests argued to not be reliable
July 2005 to December 2005	Australian Football League resistance
	BALCO court cases
	Lance Armstrong accusations and further UCI/WADA conflict
	Four-year ADRV ban considered
	Pound has a public dispute with Hein Verbruggen
	UNESCO agreement formalised
	IOC and Italy dispute over federal doping punishment in Italy
January 2006 to June 2006	National Hockey League dispute before Turin Games
	Zach Lund ADRV
	Turin scandal
	Wendell Sailor ADRV
July 2006 to December 2006	Operation Puerto
	Floyd Landis ADRV
	Justin Gatlin ADRV
	Australian Football League resistance
	Marion Jones ADRV cleared
	Altitude tents controversy
January 2007 to June 2007	Pound independence criticised again
	Floyd Landis ADRV
	Australian Football League resistance
	Beijing Olympics build up
July 2007 to December 2007	Ian Thorpe AAF
	Floyd Landis ADRV
	Pound replaced by John Fahey as WADA president
	Operation Raw Deal
January 2008 to June 2008	New human growth hormone test produced
	Credibility of John Fahey questioned
	Beijing Olympics build up
July 2008 to December 2008	Dwain Chambers ADRV appeal
	Drugs trafficking problems
	Gene doping concerns
	Concern over testing at Beijing Olympics
	IOC to retest frozen blood samples
January 2009 to June 2009	Random whereabouts drugs testing complaints
	Matt Stevens ADRV
	Lance Armstrong
	IOC sample retests
July 2009 to December 2009	The Board of Control for Cricket in India (BCCI) and WADA conflict

(*Continued*)

Date	News Stories
	Andre Agassi AAF
	Richard Gasquet AAF
January 2010 to June 2010	OOC testing concerns
	Terry Newton ADRV
	Floyd Landis accuses Armstrong of doping
	BCCI cricket still resisting
July 2010 to	Alberto Contador ADRV
December 2010	Concerns over Delhi commonwealth games
	Marijuana kept as a banned substance
	Operation Greyhound
January 2011 to June 2011	Alberto Contador ADRV
	Kolo Toure ADRV
July 2011 to	Indian 4×100 women's team case
December 2011	WADA announces partnership with GlaxoSmithKline
	National Football League dispute with WADA
	English Football Association naming players after tests dispute
	Alberto Contador ADRV
	Dwayne Chambers life ban dispute between British Olympic Association (BOA) and WADA
January 2012 to June 2012	BOA and WADA dispute over suspension lengths for Dwayne Chambers and David Millar leading into London 2012
	London lab procedures highlighted
	Alberto Contador ADRV
	Dispute between Spain and WADA
July 2012 to	WADA switches to advocating for four-year bans after BOA row
December 2012	Concerns over Kenyan doping
	Lance Armstrong found guilty
	United States Anti-Doping Agency (USADA) and UCI dispute
	Dwayne Chambers and David Millar participate at 2012 London Olympics
January 2013 to June 2013	Lance Armstrong – UCI and WADA dispute over dropped doping probe
	Operation Puerto goes on trial, and Spain linked to cover-up
	EFC case
	Kenya doping concerns
	Vijay Singh AAF
July 2013 to	EFC case
December 2013	Evidence of Russian doping
	Kenya doping concerns
	Reedie changes focus to compliance and assisting nations
	Lack of testing on Jamaican athletes
	Lance Armstrong ADRV
	Approval of four-year bans

(Continued)

Date	News Stories
January 2014 to June 2014	Lack of testing on Jamaican athletes EFC case Kenyan doping probe Chris Froome therapeutic use exemption (TUE) case
July 2014 to December 2014	Cronulla Sharks doping and Australian Sports Anti-Doping Authority (ASADA) dispute with WADA EFC case Kenya doping probe ARD documentary aired about Russian doping and first Pound investigation launched
January 2015 to June 2015	EFC case Cycling Independent Reform Commission (CIRC) report published Alberto Salazar
July 2015 to Dec 2015	EFC case Anti-Doping Association of Kenya formed Pound report findings IAAF first attempt at blocking doping report from 2011 Daegu IAAF World Championships Alberto Salazar Vitaly Mutko links to FIFA scrutinised Bulgarian weightlifters ADRV
January 2016 to June 2016	Russia and second Pound report IAAF corruption EFC case Resetting world records suggested Adidas and Nestle drop sponsorship of IAAF Maria Sharapova Ethiopian doping concerns 2012 London Olympics retrospective testing Operation Puerto blood bags released
July 2016 to December 2016	Kenyan drugs investigation via United Kingdom Anti-Doping Agency (UKAD) McLaren report IOC decision on Russian participation WADA and IOC dispute over Russian participation Fancy Bears TUE leak Bradley Wiggins TUE scrutinised Sharapova appeal successful Ethiopian doping concerns Post 2016 Rio Olympics WADA report Reedie re-election McLaren report part 2 iNADO reform suggestions
January 2017 to June 2017	Hein Verbruggen accused of corruption Concerns about Russian attempt to be compliant IOC not investigating Jamaican results

(Continued)

Date	News Stories
July 2017 to December 2017	Bradley Wiggins TUE Alberto Salazar Icarus documentary released at Sundance festival Mo Farah Icarus documentary Fancy Bears TUE Russian ban for Pyeongchang Reported Chinese doping in 1970s, 1980s and 1990s BCCI and WADA dispute
January 2018 to June 2018	Chris Froome TUE Fancy Bears release WADA emails Russian participation at Pyeongchang Winter Olympics Doping bans lifted on 28 Russian athletes Department for Digital, Culture, Media & Sport (DCMS) report on Team Sky Chris Froome AAF Kiprop AAF Guerrero AAF
July 2018 to December 2018	Froome cleared Russian Anti-Doping Agency (RUSADA) reinstatement CBD products gain popularity Cannabis legalised in Canada
January 2019 to June 2019	Baku WADA Foundation Board meeting Russia misses laboratory information management system (LIMS) data deadline Sun Yang failed test collection Sharapova returns Global Athlete launch BCCI non-compliance
July 2019 to December 2019	Mack Horton protests at Sun Yang Shayna Jack AAF Prithvi Shaw case Christian Coleman whereabouts Missing Russian data Alberto Salazar found guilty Sun Yang hearing
January 2020 to June 2020	Russia banned from Olympic sports for four years Sun Yang given eight-year suspension Weightlifting Federation corruption Christian Coleman whereabouts

(Continued)

Index

9780367540647